F

The Healing Choice

Your Guide
to Emotional Recovery
After an Abortion

Candace De Puy, Ph.D.
and
Dana Dovitch, Ph.D.

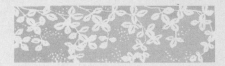

A FIRESIDE BOOK
Published by Simon & Schuster

FIRESIDE
Rockefeller Center
1230 Avenue of the Americas
New York, NY 10020

Designed by Laura Hough

Manufactured in the United States of America

10 9 8 7 6 5 4 3 2 1

Library of Congress Cataloging-in-Publication Data

De Puy, Candace.
    The healing choice : your guide to emotional recovery after an abortion / Candace
De Puy and Dana Dovitch.
        p.   cm.
    Includes bibliographical references and index.
    1. Abortion—United States—Psychological aspects.   2. Abortion counseling—
United States.   3. Post-traumatic stress disorder.   4. Abortion—Religious aspects.
I. Dovitch, Dana.   II. Title.
HQ767.5.U5D4   1997
363.46—dc21   96-47484   CIP

ISBN 0-684-83196-1

Material from *The Heroine's Journey* by Maureen Murdock © 1990 is reprinted by
arrangement with Shambhala Publications, Inc., 300 Massachusetts Avenue, Boston,
Massachusetts 02115.

The ideas, procedures, and suggestions in this book are intended to supplement, not
replace, the medical advice of trained professionals. All matters regarding your health
require medical supervision. Consult your physician before adopting the medical
suggestions in this book as well as about any condition that may require diagnosis or
medical attention.
        The authors and publisher disclaim any liability arising directly or indirectly from
the use of this book.

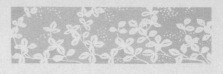

Dedication

We dedicate this book
to our parents—with love.

Lorraine De Puy and Thomas De Puy

Phyllis and Victor Dovitch

Acknowledgments

We thank you, Candice Fuhrman, Linda Michaels, Haden Blackman, Becky Cabaza, Donna Beech, Robert Gordon, Angela Bonavoglia, Jane Johnson and Connie Zweig, for guiding us through this project.

We thank you, the doctors, nurses, psychotherapists and counselors who freely gave us their valuable time and shared their knowledge: Gary Schneider, O.D., Robin Schwartz Kapper, MFCC, Gayle Pepper McClean, RN, Michael Frank, MFCC, Michael Gross, M.D., Mary Schmitz, Ph.D., Leslie Eichenbaum, Ph.D., Jenny Soriano, M.D., and Sherry Goldman, R.N. We also extend our gratitude to the many health-care workers who helped us and who wished to remain anonymous.

Soul encouragement and nurturing came from our friends and loved ones. We thank you, Janet, Pete, Kitty, Clare, Dennis, Don C., Don G., Tony, Dawn, Kathy, Mollie, Stacey, Jon, Virginia, Jerry, Stephanie, Patty C., Patty H., Aaron, Liz, Natalie, Joan, Fred, Deliane, Elizabeth, Minnie, Max and Birdie for being there unendingly.

Our sisters, Michele, Debby and Diana, we couldn't have done it without you. Our brothers, Herb and Dagoberto, thanks for being in our corner. Ric, thank you dearly for enduring the long hours away.

Most of all, we deeply thank all the women who gave us their time, their hearts, their wisdom and their insights. Your interviews served to inspire and create this book.

Contents

Introduction

Abortion is not a frivolous choice. No woman sets out to create, then terminate, a possible life; but, over the centuries, millions of women have had abortions, and millions more will continue to terminate unwanted pregnancies regardless of social, religious or legislative opinion.

This book is for any woman who feels psychological pain from her past abortion, any person who has strong feelings about abortion, any person who sees abortion as killing a child, and anybody who feels sure it is not. It is a book that lends insight and offers helpful ways to achieve post-abortion healing. This is not a book about judgment, politics or religion. It is not a book about right or wrong.

Psychological studies show that only 10 percent of the 1.6 million American women who undergo abortions every year experience severe emotional trauma following the procedure, and those women were most often psychologically unstable prior to their pregnancy. Unfortunately, most studies dismiss the other 90 percent of women as if they had no reaction whatsoever. Because the majority of women move forward with their lives, any normal grief, confusion or ambivalence they might feel is dismissed.

In reality, women who find themselves confronted with the decision to abort do not always walk away from the experience unscathed, even though they move forward with their lives. As psychotherapists, we see such women in our practices every day. Many women acknowledge a feeling of relief after their abortion, yet are understandably upset by facets of the experience that they had never anticipated. Many are distressed and unaware of the ways in which their choice has changed their lives and, sometimes, the lives of those around them. Many have been unwilling to speak of their choice in a world that is openly conflicted about abortion. Many are wracked with religious guilt and a fear that they have killed an unborn child. These reactions are not felt on the day of the abortion, but may arise over time—sometimes years later—as women reflect back upon their experience.

Beneath the clamor of the abortion debate, the quiet impact abortion has on the psychological life of the woman who makes this choice has gone unheard. There is no cultural acknowledgment that she may have struggled over her decision or felt bereaved, or that the event may have left her with pain. Thus, abortion remains a significant personal experience that is not publicly recognized, socially sanctioned or frankly shared in the way a divorce, the death of a loved one or a miscarriage might be. A woman's emotional journey from conception to termination is often left buried in her psychological underground. As she fights the external stigma, she struggles to understand her internal process, but without a charted course for healing, she has little guidance to explore, integrate or resolve her feelings.

Emotional restoration after an abortion is a unique challenge because the emotions a woman experiences are the result of a choice she made. Paradoxically, her healing journey requires yet another significant choice—a healing choice. She can either live with the unresolved memories she may have struggled to hold at bay, or she can decide to go forward, look inward and reexamine herself. To find resolution, she must acknowledge feelings and recollections, even though it is tempting to fantasize that emotions will magically resolve themselves with time.

This healing journey asks a woman to: reflect upon the circumstances and reasons for her decision; explore the emotions that led to and resulted from her abortion; examine relevant issues arising from both her family of origin and the culture in which she was raised; and realize how the overall experience may have impacted her life then and now by recognizing what she lost and what she has gained.

In an era when people are talking on national television about difficult and formerly taboo subjects, such as sexually transmitted diseases, rape and incest, it is time that post-abortion recovery be brought out from under the cloak of fear and controversy. We believe it needs to be looked at squarely and addressed frankly.

The Creation of This Book

The idea for this book arose out of our clinical relationships with female clients whose lives had been touched by an abortion. As mental health professionals, we were concerned to find how few had discussed the life-changing decision they had made. When they began to share their stories, nearly all were surprised by the depth of emotion they still felt. Even those individuals who had never experienced post-abortion pain were moved by the realization that this singular action had allowed them to create important options and changes in their lives.

To encourage our clients' healing we tried to locate helpful books they might read on post-abortion recovery. When we found that none existed, we set out to write one.

The data we collected came out of in-depth interviews with forty women who had experienced one or more abortions. The women ranged in age from eighteen to seventy-five and were from varied religious and ethnic backgrounds. More than half the women had never experienced psychotherapy. Each interview was composed of fifty-three questions regarding a woman's familial, cultural and religious background; the circumstances in her life at the time of her pregnancy and abortion; her experience of pregnancy and the abortion procedure;

and general feelings concerning shame, anger, regret, relief, the grieving process and acceptance. We also interviewed five men. The majority
of questions elicited narrative responses rather than simply "yes" or
"no" answers. In order to protect the anonymity of the participants,
their names and certain details about their lives have been changed.

In the course of our interviews we came to appreciate a unique
realm of female psychology. Again and again, we were told how a
woman's view of her abortion had changed over the course of her life
so that an abortion that appeared fully resolved in earlier years often
took on changed meaning and reappeared as a different kind of
benchmark as she matured. This aspect of post-abortion healing served
to enlighten us as to the inextricable link between a woman's emotional well-being and the changes in her body from the onset of
menstruation to the end of menopause.

As for the reactions of the women we spoke with, all of them
found comfort in the opportunity to explore the decision they had
once made. And all of them expressed hope that by sharing and
recounting their experiences, they might lend support to women like
yourself as you explore your past abortion.

Throughout the book we apply the word "fetus" to that which
was released during the abortion procedure. Some of the women we
talked to used words such as the "tissue," "it," the "baby," even the
"shrimp." For general purposes, "fetus" is the most accurate scientific
term and, unless it is a direct quote to the contrary, the one that we
will use. Our decision to do so is in no way meant to devalue the
emotionally laden experience of what, for many women, is the loss of
a baby.

What You Will Find in This Book

This book is meant to help you recount the memories of your abortion
experience, explore your emotions and gain insight and knowledge
into your own post-abortion experience. Within each chapter are

exercises to help you along your way. Some women will want to do all the exercises, others will want to pick and choose which ones are right for them, and still others will simply want to read the text. It is up to you.

The book is divided into three parts. Part 1, "The Experience," examines the history of your pregnancy in chapter 1 and your abortion in chapter 2. Your journey began the moment you conceived and your life irrevocably changed. Understanding the meaning and emotional impact of your pregnancy and abortion is the start of your healing.

Part 2, "The Aftermath," closely resembles the process of psychotherapy; we will address a variety of issues that affect post-abortion pain. In chapter 3 we will look at the ways in which you may have felt isolated, the times you may have yearned for solitude and the inevitable loss of privacy you experienced when your pregnancy was terminated. Chapter 4 tackles guilt, a normal but often challenging emotion for post-abortion women. Chapter 5 helps you explore your anger and the instrumental role it plays in the process of healing. Chapter 6 addresses the delicate realm of religious pain and conflict, and the special needs of spiritual women. Chapter 7 looks at the losses, often difficult to define, arising from your abortion and lends support as you grieve those losses.

Part 3, "Acceptance," provides extensive exercises for continued healing and closure. Chapter 8 can help you strengthen your personal insight and bring you nearer to claiming recovery. Chapter 9 speaks about acceptance—a process of continuing growth.

At the very end of the book you will find suggested reading materials and a list of resources to further your healing work. There are also suggested readings for women whose abortion recovery is complicated by other issues such as addictions and childhood abuse.

Starting the Work of Post-abortion Healing

Understanding, grieving and acceptance are at the core of post-abortion healing. But the process may not be easy. We urge you to listen to your heart and your needs every step of the way.

Feelings and memories will begin to surface as you move through the chapters and exercises. It is easy to become overwhelmed. You may need to put the book down for a little while and come back to it later, or you might find yourself wanting to shut down, numb out and take a break from your discomfort. At these times it can be better to get a closer look at your feelings than to run the other way. You do not need to rush, however, as there is no exact time frame for healing. Journal writing may be your best "healthy escape."

If, while reading this book and doing the exercises, you feel yourself struggling to deal with your emotions and memories beyond a point of comfort, stop reading, close the book and put it down. You might want to continue your post-abortion healing by reading this book with the ongoing support of a psychotherapist.

A journal can be comforting when you are filled with emotions and need a safe place in which to pour out your feelings. Journals are not for publication. Your journal is for your eyes only! Perfect grammar and correct spelling do not matter. Do not judge or critique what you write. Simply put your pen to paper and let your feelings speak for themselves in whatever way they choose. What you write is never wrong.

Pick a journal that you will want to write in. It can be an ordinary spiral notebook, a journal with an attractive cover bought at a bookstore, or perhaps a hardbound sketchbook found in an art-supply store which you can leave plain or decorate. You can fill it with thoughts, quotes, pictures, feathers, pressed flowers or anything you like. You can write in pencil or colored pen. It is all up to you.

If you have been hesitant to talk freely about your abortion with a close friend, a family member or even a counselor, your journal may become your new best friend. If you have already shared your experience with someone, your journal can serve to document the healing work you are now beginning. Throughout this book, use your journal to work through the exercises you choose to do and record your healing journey.

To begin this process, start with the following exercise.

Exercise:

Write your responses to the following questions and remember, whatever you put down is right. You do not have to write pages and pages unless you want to. Just write until you feel ready to stop.

1. How do you feel about starting this book? Are you scared, anxious, excited or feeling all kinds of different emotions?
2. What do you hope to come away with after finishing this book?
3. Have you ever kept a journal? If you have, what was that experience like? If you have never kept a journal, how do you feel about beginning one now?

Many women find it helpful to have a space in their home devoted to their post-abortion healing. If this appeals to you, think about creating a special nook in your house or apartment. It can be a space on your bureau, desk, nightstand or any place that feels right. Keep your journal there, along with this book. If there are objects that relate to your pregnancy, like a picture of the man or yourself from that time, place them there. If there is a diary you kept, letters you received, poems you have written, or works of art that you made related to your pregnancy or abortion, place them there, as well as anything you create as you read this book. This special place honors your experience and shows that you are accepting its importance in your life.

You may want to share your insights with a friend or you may want to keep the entire experience private. It is a personal decision.

As you read this book, feel free to underline passages, write notes or draw pictures in the margin.

You are headed on your path toward post-abortion healing. Your next step will take you back in time to recall the pregnancy that began your journey.

PART ONE

The
Experience

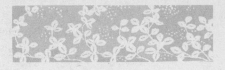

Chapter One
The Pregnancy

"Memory is history recorded in our brain, memory is a painter, it paints pictures
of the past and of the day."

—Grandma Moses

Grandma Moses: My Life's History

ed. Ottot Kallir

The journey toward resolving post-abortion pain begins with your
awareness that the decision you made to end your unwanted pregnancy
was a choice that altered the course of your life.

Women can, often with ease, recall the reasons why they chose to
have an abortion: they were not ready to have a baby; they could not
support another baby; they never wanted to have a baby; they were
pressured into terminating a pregnancy; or the fetus was diagnosed as
unhealthy. The unifying factor among these women, regardless of the
reasons behind their decision, is that few have gone on to explore or
share the experience of being pregnant, and when the unwanted
pregnancy is over, it is rarely spoken of again.

When we asked women, "What were the feelings you had when
you were pregnant?" time and again we were met with looks of

surprise. "That's a good question," they would say, or "I don't think I've ever talked about that." They then went on to list nearly identical emotional experiences: anger, guilt, shame, self-judgment, fear and depression. During their pregnancies these emotions were experienced as a barrage of undefined feelings labeled "discomfort." Afterward they were forgotten or denied. To explore them seemed too upsetting.

By recapturing your pre-abortion feelings through the following text and exercises, you may come to understand more about the meaning of your abortion.

> Nothing in life is to be feared. It is only to be understood.
> —Marie Curie

Forgotten Feelings

When an individual feels unable or unwilling to confront the emotions and memories surrounding a difficult experience, then troubling feelings or recollections may be denied, dismissed or tucked away. But painful feelings, even when suppressed, do not simply vanish. They remain dormant, waiting for a time to resurface and demand recognition.

Attempting to hold pain at bay is a response that most healthy individuals find themselves employing as they prepare to confront hurt; for example, discarding the possessions of a deceased loved one is often delayed until one feels truly ready, or discussing a troubling illness is something individuals do when they feel prepared to confront their fear. Addressing the pain of a past abortion is also often postponed until a woman feels able and ready to explore her upset.

When disturbing feelings present themselves for healing and are ignored, they will likely surface in a disguised form, such as anxiety, insomnia, addiction, depression, anger or flashbacks to the incident that first caused the hurt. To safeguard your emotional health and physical well-being, it is important to recognize and address your post-abortion discomfort if it calls for healing attention.

Exercise One:

1. For women with unresolved feelings over their unwanted pregnancy, emotions can resurface in many masked forms. Use your journal or take note of any symptoms that are familiar to you on the following list:
   - periods of depression
   - feelings of anxiety or panic
   - addictive behaviors, such as eating disorders, drug or alcohol problems, smoking, workaholism, etc.
   - stress over sexual intimacy
   - discomfort in response to some organized religions
   - tension during heated political debates over abortion
   - shame or secrecy when a doctor asks routine questions about past pregnancies
   - resistance to attending the baby shower of a good friend
   - fear of spiritual retribution
   - concern over being unable to conceive again in the future
   - fear when trying to conceive
   - unexplained feelings of depression when you do conceive
   - avoidance of newspaper and magazine articles or television programs that deal with the topic of abortion
   - the need to deeply involve yourself in movements for or against a woman's right to choose abortion
   - tension when asked, "Do you want children?" or "Do you have children?"

2. Using your journal, list other symptoms that are unique to your own experience.

> You can live a lifetime and, at the end of it, know more about other people than you know about yourself.
>
> —Beryl Markham
> *West with the Night*

Pregnancy Brings Physical Changes

Pregnancy always means physical change. If a woman has decided to abort, she must still wait for the right time for the procedure, as evaluated by a physician. While she waits for that given time, the reality of her pregnancy becomes manifest in her body. She may experience nausea, fatigue, enlarged breasts, weight gain and skin changes. These shifts speak to the event that she must confront. It is inescapable. The woman is aware of the impact of her sexual actions and viscerally bears witness to them. Pregnancy becomes a reality. Wendy shares,

> I was always conscious of how my body looked, and I was always aware that there was a life growing inside of me. It was very much in the forefront. I instantly changed.

> Each woman has different emotional and physical reactions to pregnancy, and the same woman may react differently to different pregnancies.
> —Robert Crooks and
> Karla Baur
> *Our Sexuality*

And Susan tells us,

> I felt fat! I couldn't suck in my stomach. My breasts ached—just like before I get my period—but it didn't go away. I got morning sickness six weeks into it. I was hiding crackers in my bag at work. I wasn't able to eat normal food without dashing into the bathroom.

For Laura, like many women who had already experienced pregnancy, the signs were immediate and recognizable:

> I remember quickly getting the clue that I was pregnant because there was a distinct kind of nausea that I only experience when I'm pregnant. I just knew.

But for Marianne, like some women whose bodies didn't react with obvious and immediate changes during pregnancy, the waiting period was a time of confusion. She wanted to be in denial, trying to believe that her period was just late:

> I wish there were a little dot on your face that changed color when you were pregnant, so you didn't have to go through that waiting

period! I guess some people know right away. I'm not that way. Hardly anything on me ever changes when I'm pregnant—it just feels like PMS. I just had to sit and hope that my period would come.

Exercise Two:

1. When did you first know that you were pregnant?
2. Did your body tell you immediately or did you have to wait for a missed period?
3. During the days or weeks until your abortion, what were the physical changes you experienced?

Buried Emotions

Many women who feel emotionally ill-equipped to face the serious dilemma of an unwanted pregnancy are able to deny what is happening in their bodies, even as the signs of pregnancy multiply. They talk of patiently waiting for a period, and even if they suspect a pregnancy, many still seek the refuge of denial in order to avoid frantic feelings. Wendy says,

> I waited three months before going to the doctor because I was in major denial. I was fifteen, I had no idea what was going on and I couldn't believe it could be happening to me! I really thought it was just kind of going to go away.

Janice's denial was different from Wendy's. Pregnant at twenty-two, Janice hid behind the symptoms of her eating disorder to guard against the terror of facing her pregnancy:

> I became pregnant in the midst of my eating disorder. I had been bulimic and my period was never regular, so when it didn't come I just wrote it off to my sick body. I was denying the physical symptoms that were screaming "You're pregnant!"

> I was 7 days pregnant when I called my doctor. She didn't believe me. She said it was too soon to know. I knew.
>
> —Leah
> Interview

But denial cannot change the reality of a pregnancy. Despite attempts to ignore or rationalize the symptoms away, the pregnancy ticks on until it is finally confirmed.

After the confirmation of an unwanted pregnancy, some women wrestle to find a place to direct their suffering and anger: at God; at the man involved; at themselves. A frequently cited target of anger is neglected or failed birth control. Wendy says,

> Anger is something we feel. It exists for a reason and always deserves our respect and attention.
> —Harriet Goldhor Lerner
> *The Dance of Anger*

The first time I got pregnant the condom broke. The second time I used a diaphragm with lots of jelly, and it didn't work either. I was pretty damn angry.

Even when a woman knows her anger isn't directed toward the proper place, she may still feel this powerful emotion. Jessica tells us,

My boyfriend had another girlfriend for four years before me, and they had never used birth control and never got pregnant. Because of a childhood accident, he thought he was sterile. He had never used birth control. I was young enough and naive enough to take this as a truth. So when I got pregnant, I wasn't exactly mad at him, because he didn't know. I was just mad.

Along with anger, undercurrents of fear plague women's psyches. Whom can they safely tell? Will they be punished by God? Will their relationships withstand the trauma? Anne expresses her experience with this emotion:

From the moment I found out I was pregnant I felt this very quiet fear. The whole experience was new to me, and I wasn't sure how it would all unfold. It was fear of the unknown and fear that my lover would leave me if he knew.

Vicky tells us,

I could hardly live with what was happening to me. I didn't want
other people to look at me and think of me as a possible murderer.

Sandra's fear stemmed from her religious upbringing:

I was sure that God would send me straight to hell for having
sex, getting pregnant and then planning an abortion on top of it!

Sadness and depression are also predictable responses
to the pain of an unwanted pregnancy. Author Jo Ann
Rosenfeld, M.D., writes that women are more likely to be
depressed before an abortion than afterward, when they
typically experience a sense of relief. Dr. Rosenfeld also
believes that women who continue to feel lingering sadness may be experiencing a continuation of the pain that
accompanied their pregnancy rather than any effects of
the termination.

> I'm committed to
> the idea that one of
> the few things hu-
> man beings have to
> offer is the richness
> of unconscious and
> conscious emo-
> tional responses to
> being alive.
> —Ntozake Shange
> *Black Women Writers at*
> *Work*, Claudia Tate, ed.

Andrea expresses her sadness very clearly:

I felt despair because I knew I couldn't keep it. And I knew I was
about to make a decision that I'd find really hard to live with later.

Cloe's strongest emotion was depression:

I felt very depressed. The timing was so terrible. I felt too young to
go through this. If it had happened a year down the road, I might
have been able to have a child.

Many women experience guilt, shame and harsh self-judgments
during their pregnancy. They believe that had they been more

cautious or more aware, their pregnancy could have been completely avoided.

Alta was keenly aware of her feelings of guilt. She relates,

> I felt a lot of guilt about being so stupid when I didn't want to get pregnant! I felt like a real jerk. I thought, "I want to make love without my diaphragm. I'm sure I'm going to get my period tomorrow." And that was stupid—not using all my brains. I felt really bad and ashamed for that.

> Depression—that is what we all hate.
> —Kate Millett
> *The Loony-Bin Trip*

Anne, much like Alta, had recurring feelings of guilt:

> Well, I felt guilt but I honestly can't tell you why. I was using birth control, I thought I was being very responsible. But I kept thinking, "These things don't happen unless you let them happen!" I don't feel guilty any longer, but I had to pick apart every moment of the experience to get there.

As you look back over your pregnancy, you may discover layer upon layer of buried emotions. As you uncover these feelings, you may find post-abortion pain rooted in your experience of being pregnant.

Exercise Three:

The following statements will help you sort through the emotional aspect of your pregnancy. You might discover that completing the sentences brings back the memory of one strong emotion or many emotions. You might recall difficult emotions, and you might even recall some positive ones.

1. When I thought I was pregnant, I felt . . .
2. When my pregnancy was confirmed, I felt . . .
3. The strongest feelings I remember were . . .
4. When I look back to the time I was pregnant, I now feel . . .

Unlocking your buried emotions is the first step in healing them. In order to do this work, you must be able to identify your emotions. This can be a difficult task; in order to help you do this, you will find a Feelings List in appendix one. It may be helpful to refer to it whenever you cannot name your emotions.

The Fetus

In the truest terms, a woman must face the potential for a baby during her pregnancy; thus, pregnancy can be a dark place for a woman to enter when it ends in abortion. When we asked, "How would you like us to refer to the fetus?" nearly all the women we interviewed hesitated. They usually searched for words that would separate them from that place where potential life exists:

> "I call it 'the fetus,' and in my more emotional moments I call it 'the child.' "
>
> "The bean."
>
> " 'It.' "
>
> "Fetus or tissue, I think."
>
> "Embryo—like a little peanut."
>
> "A shrimp. . . . Let's call it 'it.' "
>
> "Hmm. The egg."

The circumstances surrounding conception . . . in conjunction with a woman's psychological and social resources provide the context that will affect a woman's response to her pregnancy.

—Nancy Adler
"Psychological Factors in Abortion"
American Psychologist

If a woman were welcoming her pregnancy, she would happily speak about conceiving a baby—not an "egg," a "fetus," a "shrimp" or an "it." She would freely indulge in the abundant truths and myths of motherhood. But to call the fetus a "baby" when she is planning to abort would heighten her confusion as she psychologically pulls away from the "accident" growing in her womb.

A woman's natural sense of relatedness might now come in conflict with her inner pull toward selfhood if her present needs and goals do not include a pregnancy. To diminish this inner duality, she may call the fetus "it" rather than "baby." In the case of other women, they may truly experience the fetus as an "it"; they never believe the fetus to be a baby at all.

Exercise Four:

In your own pregnancy:

1. How did you refer to the fetus at the time of your abortion?
2. How do you refer to it today?
3. How do you feel using that word?
4. What brought you to use one particular word or phrase instead of another word?

> Pain is the great teacher . . . [it] forces us to think, and to make connections, to sort out what is what, to discover what has been happening to cause it.
>
> —May Sarton

No Bond to the Fetus

Women who feel little or no bond with the fetus, and make their decision to terminate with ease, sometimes later worry that their rejection of a pregnancy is evidence that they haven't looked deeply enough into themselves. They fear that their decision to terminate came without undue misgivings. Many of these women are relieved when, in subsequent years, they feel a maternal drive. Other women come to realize that motherhood is not something they truly desire.

Janet had no plans for children and did not feel a bond with the fetus. She initially experienced no tension in making her decision:

> I really adore children, but I never wanted a child of my own. And when I got pregnant I felt no connection to anything like "baby." I felt overwhelmed by emotion, but only because I had to go through something so unexpected and so upsetting to my body. But it was never about a baby.

Janet went on to tell us that when she turned fifty she looked at her abortion in a different light:

> My husband and I don't have any offspring—no kids or grand-children. Because I'm in menopause now, I sometimes look back on my abortion as a lost opportunity. I feel a little sad about it. At the same time, I am able to cherish all the opportunities that having no kids gave me. It is a challenge to be able to feel sad and grateful at the same time.

Jill, much like Janet, felt no bond with the fetus. She shares,

My womb filled up with something— not someone.

—Daisy
Interview

> I work with kids. I give them a great deal of myself from nine to three, and I receive a lot in return. My caring for kids is central to my life. When I accidentally got pregnant, I never felt anything about the tissue in me. To this day, I don't think of the tissue as anything [remotely similar to] a baby.

Jessica does not believe that she aborted "a baby." She felt little connection to the fetus, and even later, when the tissue became more "shrimp-like," she couldn't conjure up feelings of attachment. Jessica tells us,

> I was nineteen years old. The abortion was at about eleven weeks. I believed at that time it was only tissue. I didn't think it had any form whatsoever. But the next year my boyfriend and I went to Paris and visited a museum where many bottles of fetuses were lined up on a shelf from about six weeks to five months. I was upset when I saw a twelve-week fetus. It looked shrimp-like—nothing like a person—but it did have a form. We stood there and looked at it. We didn't talk. For quite some time after that I questioned just what a big step I

*Need ex: d
Noman who
Id'd Asbaby?*

had taken. I realized that I had to take less things for granted in my life. Maybe it was some guilt that spurred me into more awareness.

To attain personal resolution, Jessica had to work through her feelings of guilt over the abortion even though she felt no real attachment to the fetus.

Whether you felt a bond to the fetus or not, that "pregnancy" means life or potential life can be a sensitive issue. Resolving your conflict begins with a conscious awareness of any discomfort.

> . . . men try to approach the abortion decision in an abstract, intellectual way but later find themselves having to deal with feelings of hurt, guilt, or anger.
>
> —Masters and Johnson
> *Sex and Human Loving*

Exercise Five:

1. Did you experience a bond with the fetus during your pregnancy? If so, describe the bond you felt.

2. If you felt no initial fetal bond, did you develop one later? Describe when, where and how.

3. Did you feel guilt because you felt no bond?

4. Have your feelings changed over time?

The Male Partner

Unlike some lovers or brief dates who slip from a woman's memory, the man who impregnated her is permanently etched in her mind. Women may recall how they told their lovers about their pregnancy or why they withheld the news. They may recall a lack of support, sorrowful abandonment or difficult choices made together and improved relationships.

Thoughts of the "father" arouse feelings of unsettling anger in some women. Their upset, however, is not necessarily directed at a specific man. Instead, they may feel angry over the fact that they have been biologically burdened with the responsibility of birth control and have to physically deal with the ramifications of an unplanned pregnancy.

Charlotte says,

> Men don't have to experience the consequences of sex in the same
> way as women do when birth control fails.

While many women feel little lingering sorrow about their past lover or romantic encounter, they may remain baffled by the apparent lack of distress some men display during a pregnancy or after it has been resolved. The feeling that "most men don't understand what it is like to be pregnant" is frequently reported. Because the physical fact of a pregnancy is a uniquely female experience, the father cannot fully empathize.

> I don't think H. and I ever talked about that baby, and yet I don't think, given the choice all over again, that we would have done it differently.
>
> —Peter Carey
> "A Small Memorial: To the Children the Author Tried to Forget"
> The New Yorker

Some of the men we interviewed were distressed about the practical implications of a pregnancy, but were less upset about the fetus or cultural myths of fatherhood. They mentioned financial worries, feeling unprepared for fatherhood and having concerns about bringing a baby into a relationship they felt uncertain about. Other men who were already fathers did experience a connection to the fetus. For them, the decision to abort was more difficult.

Even when the man involved expresses great emotional concern over an unwanted pregnancy, symptoms of depression are rare amongst post-abortion men, suggests researcher P. Benvenuti. Those men most likely to reflect on the experience remained in relationships with their partners, already had children with their mates, or went on to have them later.

Some women feel the relief and challenge of making a joint decision with their partners. Ruth tells us,

> This was my fourth pregnancy. I already had three children. I was
> thirty-nine years old and living with my husband and children. We

had birth control, condoms, but we didn't use any because I thought I was getting my period, but actually I was ovulating. I couldn't count! My husband was very involved in the choice. He had very strong feelings that I should have an abortion.

Other women's decisions to abort are complicated by their relationship to their partner. Anne says,

> Nobody objects to a woman being a good writer or sculptor or geneticist if at the same time she manages to be a good wife, good mother, good looking, good tempered, well groomed and unaggressive.
>
> —Leslie M. McIntyre

I was engaged to someone I'd dated for four years. When we first got together he really wanted a family and so did I. Somewhere during that time he told me that he had changed his mind about having kids, but I hadn't. When I got pregnant I didn't even tell him, and shortly after my abortion I ended the relationship.

The truth that pregnancy is a different experience for women than it is for men can leave women isolated as they sort out difficult emotions regarding their mate, future relationships and feelings about the world women inhabit.

Exercise Six:

When lingering post-abortion pain, conflict, anger and sorrow are rooted in unresolved emotions over the man who fathered the fetus, a woman must unburden herself. In the past, she might have found herself having conversations in her mind where she confronted him, confided in him, sought comfort from him or revealed the abortion if she had not already told him.

If you have felt unresolved over your relationship with the man, answer the following questions as if you were writing to him:

1. Something I have never told you is . . .
2. What I want you to know now is . . .

3. This is difficult to write because . . .

4. This feels good to write because . . .

5. The most important things I want you to understand are . . .

Even when a woman receives emotional support from her mate, she walks through her pregnancy alone; it is her pregnancy, her abortion and her body. With her body pregnant, thoughts about motherhood naturally arise. Most post-abortion women entertain what impending "motherhood" should or could have meant to them.

> No woman can call herself free until she can choose consciously whether she will or will not be a mother.
>
> —Margaret Sanger
>
> *Parade*

The Myths of Motherhood

Pregnancy is "supposed" to be a happy time when a woman rejoices in her ability to create new life. She may have previously wondered, "Can I do it?" And now the answer is a resounding "Yes!" as her body explodes with the hormonal rush that alters her physical and emotional self. She is fulfilled. She beams. She radiates.

The news travels. Our mythical woman is congratulated. Gifts are bestowed upon her. She decorates a special room, the nursery. Through nine months of expectation, happiness and physical discomfort, she awaits the arrival of the bundle of joy who will complete her life.

The concept that "biology equals destiny" has been a powerful force in many women's psyches. Simply put, this notion reasons that being a woman connotes a singular mission: to bear life. It does not imply that she will not desire other challenges, such as career or travel, but these are regarded as options that she may or may not choose to explore while, according to the myth, the desire to have a child is inescapable.

Many of us have grown up with this "myth of motherhood," and some of us still believe conception will guarantee happiness, improve a bad marriage or provide a purpose for being.

This mythology is so embedded in our culture that, even when a woman is aware of it, she may still be its victim. Every woman is asked many times in her life, "Do you want children?" And should she opt for marriage, one of the first questions she gets is, "When will you have children?" Implicit in these queries is the message that wanting children and having children is a mark of normalcy.

Just as the assumption that a woman will want to bear a child is rooted in our culture's teachings, it is often considered a woman's implicit moral responsibility to exercise care and to avoid hurting others in all her relationships. She is told that giving birth is her "obligation" as a female, writes author and Harvard University Professor Carol Gilligan. The myth tells a woman that she should embrace a pregnancy as a gift and as a responsibility to take on without question, even when it is unplanned.

> . . . a woman has about thirty years of potentially fertile sex—that's a long time to go without a slip-up.
>
> —Katha Pollitt
> *Reasonable Creatures*

If a woman with an unwanted pregnancy has unconsciously internalized the absolute cultural myths of motherhood, she might take these messages, turn them back on herself as judgments and view herself as abnormal for rejecting the fetus she

Myths of Motherhood

1. I'll finally be fulfilled.
2. I'll have someone to take care of me in my old age.
3. I'll receive unconditional love.
4. There will be someone to carry on the family's bloodline.
5. I'll have someone to teach about life.
6. We'll always have happy family dinners together.
7. Holidays will be better.
8. I'll make friends with other mothers.

"should" want to care for. If a woman feels she is bad, heartless or selfish, she must question the programming she has come to live by.

Exercise Seven:

Beginning questions you can ask yourself about the effects of the culture's values on your own beliefs are:

1. Do I feel guilty when I consider having no children?
2. If I already had children at the time of my abortion or had them later, do I feel ashamed that I didn't want another?
3. Whenever I talk passionately about my work or personal interests, am I embarrassed that I don't feel as enthusiastic about children?
4. Do I think childless women are less feminine?
5. To lead a full life, is it (or was it) required that I have children?

> Necessity does the work of courage.
> —George Eliot
> *Romola*

The Unwanted Pregnancy

The concept of biological destiny begins to crumble when a woman suspects that she is carrying an unwanted fetus. The unquestioning conviction that she "should" welcome a pregnancy, no matter when it happens, is replaced by a stark reality: sexual pleasure offers the gamble—not necessarily the "gift"—of pregnancy. Whether she thinks about it or not, a woman risks meeting her reproductive potential each time she chooses to engage in sexual intercourse, from puberty to the onset of menopause.

Women also run the risk of unwanted conception when they are the victims of sexual assault. Sixteen thousand American women report abortions as a result of rape or incest each year, and those girls and women who find themselves pregnant in such a situation usually confront the "biology equals destiny" ideology.

When a woman suspects that she might have an unwanted

pregnancy, great tension and deep distress often develop. Whether she used birth control or not, she never intended to become pregnant. Now she is plagued by questions: "What am I going to do?" "How will this impact my relationship?" "Who will pay for an abortion?" "Whom will I tell?" Added to these practical concerns are her varied emotions, which may be further impacted by the hormonal upset of conception.

> Action is eloquence.
>
> —Shakespeare
> *Coriolanus*

Personal Readiness

During the days or weeks until her abortion, a woman tries to get through her daily routine, despite the stress and emotion she may be feeling. How does she get from point A to point B without falling apart, losing her job or succumbing to a deep depression?

Anne shifted into a different zone, somewhere between feeling and numbness, denial and reality:

> I felt disconnected from myself and the world. It amazes me to think that I went to work each day and actually functioned. I remember so little from that time. I was just waiting until my appointment. That's what I lived for. It helped me to avoid thinking about what was really going on.

Positioning herself in that "in-between" place was Anne's coping strategy. She planted one foot in her daily life of schedules, phone calls and normal activities, and the other foot in a private world of pregnancy discomfort and abortion planning. Only occasionally did a flood of feelings break through: in the shower, driving the car, lying in bed at night, stirring the soup. These brief "breaks" revealed the sadness and anxiety under her resolve to abort. While she felt her abortion decision was right, she largely postponed her feelings for a later time.

A pre-abortion woman rarely has the luxury of time to thoroughly assess the meaning of her pregnancy before heading into plans for termination. In her state of pregnancy and emotional turmoil, it can be difficult to systematically reason through all the details, weighing the pros and cons, to reach a plan of action. So, if she believes that abortion is her best option, she usually does it as soon as possible.

Exercise Eight:

List the reasons you ended your pregnancy.

1.

2.

3.

4.

5.

6.

If you need more space, write in your journal.

Exercise Nine:

Reflect back on the questions you have already answered in this chapter. Now:

1. Tell your pregnancy story in your journal or to a trusted friend. Begin your exploration at the beginning:

   a. How old were you?
   b. Where were you living?
   c. Who was the man with whom you conceived?

> Unwanted children have a higher incidence of physical or mental impairment, and the families of these children have a higher incidence of psychiatric disorders, educational deficiencies, criminal behavior and alcoholism.
>
> —Jo Ann Rosenfeld, M.D.
> "Emotional Responses to Therapeutic Abortion"
> *American Family Physician*

d. When did you first discover you were pregnant?

e. Did you already have children?

f. Did you want children?

g. What was your relationship to your family?

h. What was your financial status?

i. How did you feel each step of the way?

A decision to abort is only the beginning. Going into a clinic, doctor's office or hospital for the termination procedure brings a whole new set of circumstances and emotions.

Chapter Two

The Abortion

"There is plenty of courage among us for the abstract but not for the concrete."
—Helen Keller
Let Us Have Faith

As you approached the day of your abortion, feelings of turmoil may have drifted in and out of your awareness from morning until night. While striving to maintain the normalcy of daily life you may have taken unsettling breaks to make the arrangements to terminate your pregnancy. For some women, the actual abortion day is only a hazy memory. For others, every detail remains unforgettable.

A clinical abortion happens in a matter of minutes; yet any woman who has been through the procedure knows that only her physical pregnancy was terminated that quickly. Careful reexamination of your abortion experience is helpful in understanding any physical or emotional stress you may still carry from that day.

Emotional Buildup Before the Procedure

It is normal to be distressed over any invasive procedure no matter how safe, easy or efficient. Few people are comfortable having a tooth filled, blood drawn or even a tiny splinter removed. We bashfully ask, "Will it hurt?" and try to resist bolting out of the room when the hand with the needle comes toward us. Encouraging ourselves, as we would a child, we think: "Be brave," "Don't cry," "Grow up." As the anxious pre-abortion woman approaches the treatment room, she too tells herself that the relief she will feel when it is all over will be worth the tension she must now endure.

> How we remember, what we remember, and why we remember form the most personal map of our individuality.
>
> —Christina Baldwin
> *One to One*

One would be hard pressed to find a woman who would eagerly submit to an annual pelvic exam and Pap smear. An abortion takes this physical invasion countless leaps forward. It is an unexpected and unwanted crossing of boundaries. The procedure extends beyond the private territory of a woman's vagina—which usually has only been touched by lovers, physicians or her own hand—and reaches directly into her womb.

Emotional distress may be especially difficult for a very young

Abortion Facts

1. 12 percent of abortions are performed on females who are minors.
2. Abortion rates are highest in eighteen–nineteen-year-olds.
3. 60 percent of abortion women are under twenty-five years of age.
4. More than 77 percent of abortion women express a desire for children in the future.
5. 82 percent of abortion women are not married.
6. 48 percent of abortion women already have children.

woman. A clinical abortion is frequently her first encounter with the medical community and often the first time she has had a gynecological procedure. Thus, physically opening herself to the extent required for an abortion can evoke a sense of emotional crisis. Distress can be even more pronounced when it is also a woman's first experience with anesthesia. The thought of being "put out" can be as upsetting as her fear of pain.

In an ideal situation, a woman is able to choose the setting that seems best suited to her needs, the clinician who will perform the procedure and the option for anesthesia. Many women, however, find that their choices are dictated by finances or insurance coverage. Such restrictions can increase feelings of insecurity and anxiety as the abortion day approaches.

> Anxiety is essential to the human condition.
>
> —Rollo May

Clinical Settings and Security

Most hospitals, clinics and doctors' offices offer abortions in safe settings. Protestors, however, have been systematically identifying many of the locations where abortions take place. Some of these facilities are intermittently harassed by demonstrators who attempt to stop women from proceeding with their abortions, thereby creating an uncomfortable setting. Sharon had such an experience.

In 1994, after much soul-searching, Sharon and her husband sought to abort a four-month fetus diagnosed with Down's syndrome. Sharon wanted to have the procedure at the hospital where her first child had been born, but that environment, which she had found so supportive and safe during her first pregnancy, was no longer an option because the hospital refused to perform abortions after the third month of pregnancy, regardless of the reason.

Sharon's physician referred her to a local clinic to begin a three-day process for her late-term abortion. He assured her that she had nothing to fear and would be in good hands, but the experience was far from comforting:

> Each of those three days I had to go to a different location and each place was surrounded with barbed wire. I had to be buzzed in and buzzed out. Security guards were inside and outside in the parking lot. The whole thing was very secretive. On day one they wouldn't tell me where I would be on day three; they would only give me a map and directions to my next day's location. The whole time I was wondering, "Is there going to be a riot?"

Anxiety is a thin stream of fear trickling through the mind.
—Arthur Somers Roche

Sharon used a support system of "inner prayer and outward hugs" to help her through her ordeal.

Marie was in nursing school when she became pregnant in 1968. She was unmarried and determined to complete her education, and a fellow student helped her locate a doctor who would perform an abortion:

> My friend Tracy and I went to this beautifully appointed office in a very good part of town. The doctor was cold and distant. He never looked at me, and I don't think he said two words. He did some procedure, probably a D & C, and I was so intimidated and guilt ridden that I never asked a question. There was no anesthesia, no antibiotics, no painkillers to go home with. I left his office with slight bleeding that the nurse said was normal, but I started to hemorrhage in the middle of the night. I ended up in the emergency room of the teaching hospital where I was a student. It wasn't a secret any longer.

True stories like Sharon's and Marie's frighten women who may already be ambivalent about their abortion decision. Other women experience little or no inconvenience resulting from their choice of a clinical setting. Libby shares,

I went to a wonderful clinic. A nurse held my hand as the anesthesia took effect, and when I woke up, she was still there holding my hand. I felt safe and cared for.

Exercise One:

Use your journal to consider the following:

1. What kind of setting did you select? A doctor's office? A hospital? A clinic? Other?
2. How did you choose the clinical setting for your abortion? Did you have a choice?
3. How safe did you feel in the setting?
4. If you faced any threats to your physical or emotional well-being, what were they and how did they affect you?
5. List what went well on your abortion day.
6. List what did not go well on your abortion day.

> When you get to the end of your rope, tie a knot and hang on.
> —Anonymous

Coping Practices

Unpredictability can create anxiety, fear, tension and stress. As with many things in life, unpredictability also makes it impossible to anticipate the details of an abortion and plan for a positive experience. Many variables cannot be controlled, including: the mood of the clinic or office; the personality of the staff; the character of the doctor; the reliability of a woman's support system; and how she will feel on that particular day. Since the woman cannot predict the future, her coping strategies are designed to anticipate and manage negative stimuli from within and from without.

The pre-abortion woman who feels physically and emotionally fragile frequently seeks ways to minimize her confusion and anxiety on her abortion day. Because the best antidote for anxiety is information, she might use her anxiety to identify specific concerns about the day of her termination procedure: "Will I be treated well?" "Will I feel pain?" "How will I be afterward?" "What should I expect?" In considering further possibilities, she defines where she believes her anxiety originates and deals with those sources by employing self-protective coping strategies.

> One can build [her] security upon the nobleness of another person.
>
> —Willa Cather

Exercise Two:

1. What were the concerns you had on the day of your abortion?

2. List any coping strategies you consciously planned or spontaneously employed for the day of your abortion.

3. List any coping strategies you wish you had employed to help you on that day.

Reaching Out for Support

Feeling the cumulative tension of contending with her pregnancy, her emotions, perhaps her lover and parents, her finances, her work schedule and the termination procedure, a woman may reach out to others on the day of her abortion. She may choose to bring a trusted family member, friend or partner with her for support. Megan was accompanied by her mother and boyfriend. Relying on them for comfort allowed her to experience her fear in a healthy way:

> Oh, I was a mess. I cried from sheer stress and dread of the unknown. There is nothing like a good support system to make you feel safe enough to fall apart. I actually think that was good for me. I let it all out.

A woman may find herself turning to the clinic's professionals for understanding, but she cannot always count on receiving compassion from the staff. While doctors, nurses and others involved are in no position to pass judgment on a woman's actions, in reality, an occasional staff member may not be in favor of her decision to abort. Or staff members may be supportive of her decision, but might appear distant due to overwork or the intentional maintenance of professional boundaries meant to keep them disengaged from her personal life.

Overall, it appears that women who choose to bring a trusted confidante fare better than those who count on the clinical or hospital staff for comfort.

Exercise Three:

1. Did someone accompany you to your appointment? Who?
2. How did you make the choice to bring someone?
3. How did you make the choice of whom to bring?
4. Describe the ways in which the support or lack of support you received on that day helped or hurt you.

> We do not so much need the help of our friends as the confidence of their help in need.
> —Epicurus
> "Vatican Sayings"

Secrecy

While women feel entitled to share everything about their pregnancies, from Lamaze classes to episiotomies, few women feel free to swap abortion stories. No one asks about abortion, as they would about birth: "Gee, are you excited?" or "So, how was it?" When a woman recalls her abortion as abusive, difficult or sad, it often remains a secret tale of hardship.

If you kept silent about your termination or disclosed your decision to only a trusted few, you might have believed that speaking openly about your abortion would have increased your distress. If you remained silent, you might have felt that disclosing your plans would have caused you to feel judged by others, forced you to justify your actions, made you question your decision to abort when it was difficult to come by, or in any way threatened your independence.

The words "secret" and "abortion" have long gone together. Before abortions were legal in the United States, women were forced to seek "back alley" abortions. Some doctors performed abortions on the sly, but many women had to leave the country in search of a doctor or midwife to aid them. The stories women relate are alarming.

Deneen tells us that in 1967, at the age of eighteen, she was entering her junior year of college when she became pregnant. Because abortion was still illegal, there was no question as to her need for secrecy:

> What is told in the ear of a man is often heard 100 miles away.
> —Chinese proverb

I flew to El Paso. Four other girls and I were picked up in a taxi that took us to a clinic in Mexico. The people were nice, but it was dark and dank—not up to American standards. We were told we had to spend the night. We had tubes up in us to dilate our cervixes and had to stay that way all night. It was very, very painful, with severe cramping. We could only have aspirin. I remember lying on my side, tossing and turning. I just tried to get through the night. One girl couldn't handle the pain. She was screaming and crying. They left an old Mexican woman with us as a nurse but she couldn't speak English. Finally the doctor was called and gave this girl extra medication. At five or six o'clock in the morning, they came in. They got her first. I was third. They put me out and did a D & C. We woke up in a recovery area, got dressed, got in a taxi headed for the airport, and the border police stopped us. We had to stand against a building. The taxi driver paid off the cops; he made a deal with them. We were sweating because we thought we'd have to go to jail.

Although Deneen's fears permeated every aspect of her experience, she had a strong need to complete her college education and a powerful drive to be successful in her chosen field. Deneen recalls always possessing feelings of moderate to high self-esteem which, at the time of her abortion, were running concurrently with feelings of shame. Yet shame could not stop her from pursuing her goals, and she sought to safeguard her aspirations through a secretive abortion.

Deneen's character traits are mirrored in the 1988 National Longitudinal Study of Youth. Researchers Russo and Zierk took a sampling of 5,295 women between 1979 and 1987, examining several factors, including the relationship between abortion and self-esteem. They found that girls and women who had experienced abortions had "higher global self-esteem compared with women who had never had an abortion."

Although many girls and women may have normal feelings of tension, anxiety, shame or grief surrounding an abortion, their decision to end a pregnancy stems from a need to continue in their chosen life direction. A woman's decision to remain secretive during and often after the abortion procedure is not necessarily an indicator of shame or low self-esteem. It may be her best way of protecting the healthy self-esteem she already has.

> Silence is as full of potential wisdom . . . as the unhewn marble of great sculpture.
> —Aldous Huxley
> *Point Counter Point*

Emotional Shutdown

While a woman sits in the waiting room on her abortion day, she may look for a way to be emotionally absent. Her need to disconnect from the experience allows her to cope with the fact that she has chosen to terminate the fetus.

A near emotional shutdown, as common as it may be, is a response that directly conflicts with a woman's natural internal drive toward relationship to others—even when the "other" is fetal tissue. Psychotherapist and author Naomi Ruth Lowinsky believes that whether a woman views a fetus as life or potential life, she knows, on some deep level, that an "abortion is not merely a medical procedure. It is the [taking] from the womb of our own flesh and blood. It is a sacrifice of life, hopefully for life." The sheer intensity of this fact may result in a woman's need to emotionally separate from herself, the fetus and the abortion. She does not want to be present for the separation of "that something" from within her; thus, there is often a pressing need to get through the abortion with as little awareness as possible.

In a desire for complete psychological shutdown, it is not uncommon for women to request total anesthesia. Trish tells us,

> I really wanted drugs. I did not want to be awake. I wanted to close my eyes, have it done, wake up and have it be over with. I didn't want to experience anything that resembled a birth experience, since, as a mother already, I knew what that was. So I called different places to find out if they would put me out or not. When I found the clinic that said it was an option, I signed up for it. I waited in a long line. It was lonely. I felt very alienated. I couldn't wait till it was over. I was glad to go under and have it be done.

> Inside myself is a place where I live all alone and that's where you renew your springs that never dry up.
>
> —Pearl Buck
> *New York Post*

As Trish created a sense of distance from herself, from the other women waiting for their turn and from the professionals there to see her through the abortion experience, she also unwittingly created a paradox. Her protective boundaries uncomfortably isolated her even as they shielded her. Like Trish, other women expressed the same desire to distance themselves from the experience:

> It was: close the door, put me out, no connection.
>
> —Sara

> I didn't know anything about abortions before this except that I had a choice of being awake or put out, and I wanted to be put out.
>
> —Mary

The desire to be absent from the abortion experience was described by Los Angeles gynecologist Dr. Jenny Soriano as a "constructive medical concern." Dr. Soriano recommends sedation, as she believes that it safeguards a woman not only from physical pain, but from the potential of increased emotional pain as well.

Tina had her abortion at a clinic where anesthesia was not available. Although certain that at seventeen years of age she was too young to raise a child, she still felt sad that this "potential child was not going to be." She was awake during her abortion, and her physical pain became emotional anguish—something from which she wished she could have absented herself. She says,

> My abortion felt like a punishment. "You've done something very wrong and now you're going to pay." I felt pretty bad. There was no turning back for me. I had to go forward, and I couldn't stop feeling punished.

While women have yet to report absolutely foolproof coping strategies, a pre-abortion woman hopes that the abortion procedure will not add to any emotional despair she has felt since the confirmation of her pregnancy.

> After all, it is those who have a deep and real inner life who are best able to deal with the irritating details of outer life.
>
> —Evelyn Underhill
> *The Letters of Evelyn Underhill*

Healthy Coping Alternatives

No single coping mechanism works best for women who experience distress on their abortion day. But women who report the least amount of emotional aftermath describe common threads: self-knowledge, a realistic assessment of their resources and a truthful evaluation of the people and the supportive elements that exist around them.

The women we spoke with recalled things that helped them on that day, such as proper nutrition, extra rest and employing relaxation techniques. They used helpful coping strategies such as carrying a favorite pillow, bringing an audiocassette player with calming music, wearing comfortable clothes, such as sweats and sneakers, or praying off and on throughout the day. Amy shares,

> During the entire process I was chanting the words I use in yoga class to help me keep calm and not become overwhelmed by my sadness.

Janet concentrated on preparing herself to expect the unexpected:

> I didn't anticipate that every nurse would be attentive, that the paperwork would be enjoyable or that a cold operating room would be comfortable.

> Our feelings are our most genuine paths to knowledge.
>
> —Audre Lorde
> *Black Women Writers at Work* Claudia Tate, ed.

As you approached the day of your abortion your primary concern was probably to get through it and move on. Whether you rallied a support system or went to your abortion by yourself, whether you received support from the professional staff or felt alone, or whether you employed active coping strategies or toughed it out by sheer willpower, you survived a difficult experience.

It is important to recognize the inner strength it required to see yourself through your abortion. Giving yourself credit is, unfortunately, also a prime opportunity for your inner critical voices to tell you that "credit is the last thing you deserve." These voices might tell you that your fear and guilt were a punishment for your choice to abort. Recognizing and addressing these voices is another challenge and something that will be worked on throughout this book.

Exercise Four:

1. List the judgmental "barbs" your inner critical voices, or "inner critic," threw at you on your abortion day. Examples might be: "You should have gone to a less expensive clinic," "You shouldn't have gone alone," "You are too whiny."

2. Which ones still sting today?

Emotional Responses

The most common emotional reaction immediately after an abortion, even as women awake from sedation, is "relief," according to nurse practitioner Gayle Pepper McClean. McClean believes that a woman's awareness that the procedure is now over, coupled with her knowledge that she can now move forward with her life, is responsible for this sense of well-being.

Physician Gary Schneider tells us that after most gynecologically related surgeries—including births and hysterectomies—it is not uncommon for women to cry in the recovery room. And many women relate finding themselves in tears following their abortion. When asked what they felt, they invariably say, "Relief and a lot of other emotions, but most importantly, I just needed to cry." No doubt, there are complex internal and external forces behind a woman's post-abortion tears.

> A ruffled mind makes a restless pillow.
> —Charlotte Bronte
> *The Professor*

Several research studies, including one conducted by Nancy E. Adler of the University of California, San Francisco, have correlated some degree of post-abortion discomfort with the treatment a woman receives at the time of the procedure. The more stress she encounters, the greater the likelihood that she will have lingering negative aftereffects. She must then face not only the wounds from terminating an unwanted pregnancy, but the additional turmoil caused by the circumstances surrounding the procedure intended to resolve her problem. Such detrimental factors could include the behavior of the health-care providers, an imposing sterile room with unfamiliar medical instruments, waking up in recovery alone, or stressful elements in the surrounding environment, such as protesters outside the clinic.

When a clinical abortion is conducted with concern for a woman's well-being, the woman can more easily process her feelings. Laura reports that a positive environment actually hastened her emotional recovery:

I elected to have it done with a local anesthetic. I was completely awake for the procedure, and it was gentle in every respect. The staff was really crackerjack, and there was a nurse with me at all times. The doctor was about as gentle as I could imagine him being. And all the follow-up was really nurturing.

Today, Laura carries no undue emotional discomfort or trauma associated with that abortion day.

> Explore thyself. Herein are demanded the eye and the nerve.
>
> —Henry David Thoreau
> "Conclusions"
> *Walden*

Although many women feel relief immediately following their abortion, relief may be only one aspect of the complex emotions generated by the overall abortion experience. Women sometimes begin to have uncomfortable emotions months or years after the actual procedure. They may become bewildered by this next wave of feelings and find themselves reticent to look at them. These emotions are articulated as confusion, guilt, anger, sadness and anxiety.

Recollections of the event eventually return, for a clinical abortion does not terminate one's memories. Many women, now at peace with their past abortions, told us that their abortions were only truly complete once the meaning within such memories had been realized and their feelings had been resolved.

Exercise Five:

1. What were your emotions immediately after your abortion?
2. What were they later in the day? That week? The next month? Now?
3. What kinds of thoughts or beliefs emerged or changed through that time? Examples might be: "I felt oddly depressed but relieved at the same time," "I was scared to have sex," or "I won't depend on a man to use birth control again."

Backlash Emotions and Behaviors

When emotions are denied, cut off or held at bay, they will most likely return at another time in an exaggerated or disguised form. These are backlash emotions, which trigger secondary feelings and can cause unhealthy behaviors detrimental to women.

Addictions to alcohol, drugs, food, spending, work and sex sometimes plague the person who has neglected exploring and growing from an emotional experience. Addictions offer immediate emotional escape and a false sense of control. The woman who has not confronted her complex emotional life prior to her abortion, and finds that these aftermath emotions are difficult to untangle, may painfully endure or outright mask her past abortion feelings with an addiction.

Perhaps she drinks to ease the pain of her abortion and all the other hurts beneath it. Perhaps she binges when anxious and vomits to regain control. In some instances, she tries even harder at school or on the job to prove that she is strong rather than the careless, out-of-control female she fears herself to be. Maybe she abstains from sex in an unconscious or misguided attempt to regain a sense of innocence, or maybe she has sex with more men because this behavior punishes her while dulling her pain for a time.

> Girls are taught from childhood that any exhibition of sexual feeling is unwomanly and intolerable; they also learn from an early age that if a woman makes a mistake it is upon her and upon her alone that social punishment will descend.
>
> —Mary Scharlieb
> *The Seven Ages of Woman*
> 1915

Lydia's long-standing conviction that she had to be a "perfect person" in order to deserve respect collided with reality when she found herself with an unwanted pregnancy. Rather than accept herself as normal for being imperfect, Lydia quickly branded herself as a failure. Later, her post-abortion pain erupted in the disguised form of body image problems and an eating disorder:

> I was having real self-esteem problems before my abortion. Even though I was a straight "A" student, I never felt any pride. Getting

pregnant was a nightmare. It just proved my worst fear: "You aren't perfect." Anyway, I developed anorexia shortly after my abortion, but I never connected the two. I disowned my body. I became an eighty-pound skeleton. A totally non-sexual non-woman. I lost my breasts, I lost my period. I lost any mark of being "female." The really sad part is that anorexia made me feel better about myself and very safe because without a period I couldn't get pregnant.

> Compassion for myself is the most powerful healer of them all.
>
> —Theodore Isaac Rubin

Lydia sought to deny her imperfect humanness. Her misguided attempt to suppress her sexual urges and seemingly regain an image of perfection through the total control of food resulted in anorexia. Only after she claimed her normal human flaws and released herself from the pursuit of toxic excellence could Lydia heal her wounded self-esteem and post–abortion pain.

Growing up, there was no open communication about sexuality in Wendy's home; yet, she was an adolescent who came into sexual awareness at a very early age:

I wish we had really talked in my family. I wish my parents had talked to me about sex. I wish my mother was comfortable talking about getting birth control for me because I was sexually active at fifteen. I just was. I was one of those kids that became interested in sex and my body and exploring that at a much younger age than a lot of kids. I had the body of an older girl too. I had breasts when I was eleven. I got my period when I was twelve. All this happened for me sooner. I wish my mother had been comfortable talking about that. But she wasn't.

When Wendy became pregnant at fifteen she felt unable to reach out to her parents for support, fearing they would judge her. She waited a full three months into her term before secretly having a pregnancy test and an abortion.

Wendy's emotional backlash caused her to brand herself as a "bad girl" who had poor judgment, just as her parents had always told her:

My pregnancy and abortion affected me in my schooling, they affected me in my life and in my choices. They started a very destructive phase in my life that continued for many years. "See, all those terrible thoughts you had about yourself are true! You're not being a very good girl getting yourself knocked up. You're going to end up with some beer-drinking idiot in a trailer park, and your life will amount to nothing!" I think that's part of the reason I never thought college would ever be possible for me. It was almost too good for someone like me. So, I'm glad that I worked through a lot of that. And I did get my degree!

> Keeping a stiff upper lip is one thing; being able to connect to our own reality in our own situation is another.
>
> —Marion Woodman
> *Addiction to Perfection*

Since Wendy had labeled her feminine sexual nature as something dark and objectionable, the reality of her pregnancy and abortion only served to intensify her negative self-concept for several years.

Eventually, through conscious self-scrutiny, Wendy came to understand that her abortion had inadvertently symbolized the negative opinion she held of herself. Sex was not discussed in her childhood home because it was deemed wrong, and, therefore, as a sexual young woman she viewed herself as damaged goods. When she became pregnant, she felt that the "bad girl" in her was finally being punished. As Wendy healed, she began to value previously disowned parts of herself. She realized that her sexual nature was not "bad," even though it had been labeled so by the authority figures who surrounded her. By owning her sexuality, she learned how to manage it and accept herself.

In therapy, women tell stories of their wounded lives and fractured female identities. As they turn inward and investigate each thread of their lives, they sob in recognition of the deep "feeling self" they have abandoned. Slowly, patiently, and with gradual insight, they begin to find strength. Then, when they recount their pasts, including their abortion memories, they realize why they shut down; why they felt abused; why they abused themselves; why they labeled themselves; why they felt hurt, numb, sad and enraged.

There are places and moments in which one is so completely alone that one sees the world entire.

—Jules Renard

Journal, December 1900

Exercise Six:

1. In what ways might unhealed pain over your abortion have shown itself? Examples might be: not dating for years, loss of jobs, dislike or fear of sex, sentimentality over television commercials.

2. Did you face addictions after your abortion? If so, describe them.

To understand and resolve the powerful feelings resulting from the abortion day requires responsibility and commitment. An abortion ends a physical pregnancy, but it also opens new issues as a woman enters the next stage of the experience.

In the following chapter, we will explore the post-abortion experiences of separation, solitude and isolation. They can serve positive ends or they can cause additional problems, and they can begin the moment a woman first suspects her unwanted pregnancy and continue to the present day.

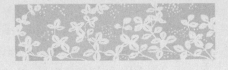

PART TWO

The
Aftermath

Chapter Three

Separation, Solitude and Isolation

"She would not exchange her solitude for anything. *Never again to be forced to move to the rhythms of others.*"

—Tillie Olsen

Tell Me a Riddle

Many politically pro-life women have had abortions, while many pro-choice women have not. Many orthodox, reform and nonreligious women have had abortions. Many have not. Neither your political stance nor spiritual beliefs can reveal your personal history—only the telling of the event can. And, as our culture is adamantly divided on the subject of abortion, despite its legality, most women choose to protect themselves with forms of privacy, solitude and isolation, before, during and after their termination.

Pregnancy separates and sets a woman apart from other people in her life. While it may impact those closest to her, it remains a profoundly personal experience. It cannot be precisely understood by any other woman nor fully appreciated by any man. When a pregnancy is welcomed, it can be acknowledged, shared and celebrated publicly; in this way pregnancy becomes a positive experience.

Like the woman who bears life, the woman who plans to abort a fetus also experiences separation from others. But whereas the woman planning to bear life may revel in her separateness, the woman moving toward abortion can experience separateness as either a trigger for emotional growth or an isolating prison.

A woman whose pregnancy is unwanted experiences separation in a private manner. She rarely exercises her right to free speech, as the culture's biases can seem forbidding. Communication with her family may be unreliable and her personal support systems weak.

> We're all in this together—by ourselves.
>
> —Lily Tomlin

Whereas chosen privacy and solitude can soothe a woman in times of emotional overload and distress, enforced isolation can spell trouble if she is in need of psychological support but cannot find it. Understanding the positive elements of solitude and recognizing the destructive triggers leading to painful isolation can enhance healing strategies.

Normal Feelings of Separateness

The first inkling of uncomfortable separation from the mainstream occurs when a woman initially suspects she has conceived an unwanted pregnancy. Understandably, she immediately feels she is dealing with a serious "problem," rather than a planned "blessing," and her emotional state radically changes. She moves through her days fearing that

SEPARATION	=	during pregnancy, abortion and post-abortion feeling different from others. A natural state.
SOLITUDE	=	a private emotional space wherein a woman processes her inner thoughts and feelings
ISOLATION	=	a place of emptiness and anguish in which a woman cannot synthesize her inner life.

"something" enormously significant and out of her control may be occurring within her body; and she knows that if this "something" is confirmed, it will irrevocably change her life.

When an unwanted pregnancy is certain, a woman separates even further and slips into a private psychological dimension. She may desire to share the information of her pregnancy as a way to seek emotional support, but finding someone who will listen with an open mind is not always possible. Even more impossible may be for the woman to understand and articulate her own emotions in order to communicate at all. Under the weight of emotional and physical shock she may choose to remain silent.

Some women feel that their decision to remain silent during their pregnancy and abortion functions for them in constructive ways. These women inevitably demonstrate a great deal of self-knowledge and possess inner "tools" to help them along their journey, such as an awareness of their needs and the ability to process their own feelings. Armed with a strong sense of autonomy, they sort through who they are and what they need without experiencing undue self-directed criticism or guilt.

> Man can be defined as the animal that can say "I," that can be aware of himself as a separate entity.
>
> —Erich Fromm
> *The Sane Society*

Rarely is a woman unquestioningly secure in her decision to abort a fetus. And rarely is she unaware that her decision might be met with disapproval. Thus, she often struggles to hear the true voice deep within her psyche that will define her core needs and help to direct her toward making a decision that she believes is "right," regardless of what others might believe. If she is able to clearly understand her reasons for terminating her pregnancy, before the abortion day, she may have an easier time accepting her past decision in years to come.

Cynthia always felt positive about herself as a person, but sometimes struggled with her past decision to abort. Even with the occasional discomfort, she believes that she did what was right at the time:

I felt torn apart when my pregnancy was confirmed. Over and over again, I kept looking inside for what I needed to do for myself. I knew I'd be terminating a fetus to choose for myself. I decided to abort so I could finish school and start my career. Right after I graduated, I was overcome with guilt. I got really confused. It took therapy and a lot of postponed tears to remember that the "sophomore me" aborted—not the graduate. Only then did I feel finished with my abortion. I realized, for the first time, how responsible I am for my own life. I also realized how responsible I'd be for a baby I didn't want.

> Alone, alone, oh! We have been warned about solitary vices. Have solitary pleasures ever been adequately praised?
>
> —Jessamyn West
> *Hide and Seek*

The magnitude of a decision such as Cynthia's, made privately and through investigation of her truest needs, is described by author Carol Gilligan: "In its simplest construction, the abortion decision centers on the self. The concern is pragmatic and the issue is survival. The woman focuses on taking care of herself because she feels that she is all alone."

Embracing aloneness as an opportunity for growth, especially during a time of extreme stress, may seem like an awesome challenge. But the experience of being alone, if only chosen for a brief time, can provide a woman with the emotional solitude in which to define her truest needs, desires and beliefs. Without the influence of others, she can thoughtfully look at her circumstances and point herself in the direction she must go.

The Healing Realm of Solitude

To feel separate from others in a time of psychological stress and serious decision making can be a natural response, but it is not always the best one when there are supportive resources available. Many psychotherapists believe that individuals who choose to isolate themselves from others in times of hardship are employing an unhealthy coping strategy. These individuals, we are told, would be better off seeking the company of others to avoid the depression that may develop out of that aloneness. This is not, however, always true.

Seeking separation, even when there are supportive resources available, is not always destructive. Separation is positive as long as it resonates with your desire to carve out a private emotional space in which to sort through your feelings and gain insight. This type of active, rather than forced, separation is called "solitude."

Psychoanalyst Anthony Storr suggests that in the privacy of solitude a person is able to evaluate her life and her choices. In solitude she comes to know herself and can define the decisions that she must make independently of others' invasive opinions and expectations. In short, solitude can allow a woman the space and time to think.

> What a commentary on our civilization, when being alone is considered suspect. . . .
> —Anne Morrow Lindbergh
> *Gift from the Sea*

Susan used her solitude to reflect on her life, her family and the man involved in her pregnancy:

> Alone, I wrestled with a lot of conflicting feelings. One moment my decision would seem clear, and the next, I felt caught in a mess of emotions. I recall wondering what my existence would be like if I had a baby. And as I considered all my planned personal goals, I imagined how a baby would affect my long-term opportunities. Would having a child be worth giving up most of my dreams? Would having a child be worth changing the life I desired?

With the clock ticking, and after a great deal of conscious consideration, Susan decided that terminating her pregnancy was painfully right for her.

Some women have the problem of an overattentive lover or

friend. At such times, they may be unable to get the solitude they require in order to hear their own hearts. Telling such a confidante that "alone time" is required is essential.

In solitude, women sort through a rush of emotions, thoughts and opinions. These may take the form of inner voices resembling a parent, clergy member, lover or other influential person. Like a committee in her mind, the voices talk to her. In whispers or shouts they give options, suggestions, "shoulds" and warnings. Although they sometimes swell into a psychological rumble, which makes it difficult to decipher each voice clearly, women are able to synthesize their truest inner voice and garner clear insights.

> Language has created the word "loneliness" to express the pain of being alone, and the word "solitude" to express the glory of being alone.
>
> —Paul Tillich

However, when a woman cannot find her way through her confusion to hear her deepest inner voice, her positive experience of solitude can degenerate into debilitating isolation.

Isolation

According to author and psychotherapist Maureen Murdock, when a woman descends to the inner regions of herself, she may experience an "incredible sense of emptiness, of being left out, shunned, left behind, without value. She may feel homeless, orphaned, in a place of in-between," and she will remain so if she is unable to resurface from her private search without some insight and clarity about her needs. She may be left in isolation with her tumultuous inner voices, her anguish and her growing problem.

If a woman makes a decision to abort, but on the deepest inner level remains in that place of "in-between," she may become depressed. An essential step in her post-abortion recovery is the recognition and examination of the debilitating voices that hold her hostage in that "in-between" place.

Ellen, who found out about the interviews for this book through her friend Melanie, had told no one about an abortion she had had eleven years ago until a week before our meeting with her. Ellen reveals,

> When my friend told me she talked to you about her abortion, she cried. I freaked. No one had ever talked to me about their abortion before. I couldn't believe she was telling me or you. And I couldn't imagine talking to you myself. But then she told me that although her boyfriend knew, way back when, she felt a thousand times better being able to hear herself talk and see you there understanding her feelings. It never occurred to me that I could talk about my abortion or that I could air my secret. So I called her the next day. This scared me a lot. It took me about four hours to dial the number. I told her that I still felt bad about my abortion. We talked and talked, and I realized that I wasn't alone. I don't know where to go with all this yet. This past week, I've just kept talking to Melanie.

> Loneliness and the feeling of being unwanted is the most terrible poverty.
> —Mother Teresa
> *Time* magazine

Ellen has recently taken the first steps away from her debilitating isolation. Her previous decision to be secretive kept her from fully experiencing and knowing the emotions surrounding her abortion, defining their significance and understanding their meaning in her life. In the months or years ahead, Ellen's work is to come to terms with her abortion through self-scrutiny and self-compassion.

Depression lifts and recovery progresses as you decode the messages from your inner voices and listen anew to the reasons you chose an abortion. But recognizing these inner voices, identifying their sources and evaluating their worth can be complicated. We are not born in a vacuum, but rather in the context of powerful cultural and family messages, all of which come together in complex ways to form our "inner voices."

Exercise One:

As you review the experience of your pregnancy and abortion, you might recall a conscious feeling of separation. The impact this feeling had upon you, whether it led to a sense of solitude that was healing or to lonely isolation, has probably influenced your post-abortion healing.

Consider the following questions:

> I grow lean
> in loneliness,
> like a water lily
> gnawed by a
>   beetle.
> —Kaccipettu Nannakaiyar
> Indian poet

1. Do you remember welcoming quiet times in which you were able to sort through your thoughts and emotions? What quiet times have you taken since your abortion?
2. Did you feel all alone or were there others whom you believed you could turn to for support? What, if any, support have you reached out for since your abortion?
3. Who were those others before, during and after your abortion?
4. Did you experience the influence of others' voices and opinions in your mind?
5. Who represented those other inner voices? Friends, family, your lover, clergy? What were they telling you?
6. Were they helpful inner voices or voices of conflict? How were they helpful? Were they hurtful?

The Effects of the Culture and Family

Psychotherapists believe that powerful outer influences add to the inner voices, which determine the decisions we make in life and our feelings about those decisions. Ideas espoused by others that truly fit with our genuine character are internalized and become synthesized with our own beliefs. Unfortunately, however, unhelpful ideas and adverse opinions can also be internalized. These can become detrimental to us if we do not recognize them and change them in ourselves. They are also detrimental when they cause us to give up the personal decisions that may be right for us.

Cultural Stigmatization

Women who cannot find a path out of their internal confusion often yearn to share their distress with others who might lend comfort and insight. Sadly, their yearning is not always fulfilled.

Many women fear reaching out, having already discovered that some of the negative inner voices that taunt them are rooted in the world around them—a world that largely shuns abortion and celebrates pregnancy. Leah told us,

> I look outside myself for guidance, but I find confusion. Then I look within myself and see a mirror of that very same confusion. Or is it the other way around? I can't tell if I feel bad about my abortion or if it is the world that is telling me that I should feel bad. It forces me into secrecy, and there I live alone.

So lonely am I
My body is a float-
    ing weed
Severed at the
    roots
Were there water
    to entice me,
I would follow it, I
    think.
    —Ono no Komachi
    Japanese poet

Terry Nicole Steinberg, a psychological researcher, has found that women like Leah often remain silent because they are concerned about social stigmatization. Says Steinberg, "If a woman could view her abortion as she views a miscarriage, as a sad event involving loss, instead of a politically and morally volatile decision, post-abortion trauma would likely decrease."

In light of Steinberg's observation and the unstable political climate, it is easy to understand why so many women have chosen to remain silent when confronted with an unwanted pregnancy. Some of the women in our interviews told us that the guilt they felt over their past terminations abated only following the legalization of abortion in 1973. As the "voice" of society changed, these women were able to internalize that new voice and transform their personal belief systems.

Living in a culture so obviously at odds regarding abortion, and witnessing the conflicting displays of compassion and violence in the face of this issue, a woman may suppress any urge to constructively share her abortion. In one study, conducted by A. Speckhard, as many as 89 percent of the women surveyed feared that other people would find out about their abortions. A woman, therefore, begins to question whether her psychological needs can ever be met in the outer world. She feels abandoned by the culture she lives in and fears the repercussions of sharing her personal story because it is controversial. As one woman succinctly stated, "My abortion is not something I shout from the rooftops."

> Wherever there is a crowd there is untruth.
>
> —Søren Kierkegaard

Poignantly sensitive to the cultural climate, many women seek a private emotional path. For better or worse, they opt for silence rather than engaging in conversations that might spark external arguments and internal debates over right and wrong. In this way, a pre-abortion woman frequently hopes to be able to proceed with her plan, and a post-abortion woman hopes to avoid heightened feelings of shame, guilt or remorse.

Exercise Two:

1. How does the culture you live in feel about abortion?
2. Did cultural pressures and opinions influence your decision to share or not to share your abortion experience?
3. If so, are you comfortable with that?

The Impact of the Family

Cultural approval may be a less critical need for a woman if there is some degree of support in her family and personal life. All too often, however, she is accustomed to an environment that either suppresses genuine emotional communication or reacts with unwarranted drama when problems arise. Her learned response may be to choose silence in order to avoid more stress, even at the risk of increased isolation.

Marianne had experienced destructive "help" resulting in isolation. At nineteen years of age, while living with her parents, she told them she was pregnant and planning an abortion:

> My mother's reaction was alien and peculiar. She was so upset. I had no idea she'd react that way. During the abortion planning I was aware that she was more upset than I was. It was confusing for me as a young woman because I wanted some help. I was lying in the hospital, about to go into the operating room, and I thought, "Wait, I'm the upset one. I shouldn't have to worry about her feelings."

> ... women in some instances deliberately choose isolation to protect themselves against hurt.
>
> —Carol Gilligan
> *In a Different Voice*

Marianne was still living at home when, at twenty-three, she became pregnant again. Having regretted sharing her first abortion decision, she decided to withhold the fact of this pregnancy from her parents. Silence, she believed, was the safest choice:

> I wanted my parents to react supportively during my first abortion, but my wish had no bearing on how they responded. They were both horrific. Because of that lesson, I chose not to tell them the second time. I protected myself from having to deal with their stuff on top of my own.

Marianne chose not to add a family crisis to her pregnancy crisis. Instead, she confided in a friend and in her sister, both of whom were better able to help her weigh her needs, come to a decision and plan for her abortion.

Exercise Three:

1. How does your family feel about abortion?
2. How might familial pressures and opinions have influenced your decision to share or not to share your abortion experience?

3. How might familial pressures and opinions have an effect on you now?

With or without the influence of cultural and family resources, a woman may constructively share her experience and avert unwanted silence by asking for professional support.

> Cultural constraints condition and limit our choices, shaping our characters with their imperatives.
>
> —Jeane J. Kirkpatrick
> Speech

Asking for Professional Support

For some women, counseling provides the only avenue for averting unwanted isolation, while other women feel that it broadens their support network and enhances their

Important Considerations When Looking for a Professional Counselor or Therapist

1. Credentials. Check to see if the therapist is licensed or is still in training.
2. Is she affordable?
3. Is a male or female counselor best for you?
4. Is she experienced with women's issues?
5. To find an unbiased therapist you might:

   a. ask a trusted minister, pastor, rabbi, doctor or friend;

   b. call Planned Parenthood;

   c. inquire if the therapist is unbiased before you see her.
6. When you meet her, ask yourself:

   a. Am I comfortable with this person?

   b. Can I trust this person?

   c. Do I feel judged by this person?

   d. Do I feel respected by this person?

   e. Is this person truly listening to me?

   f. Do I think this person is pushing her ideas on me? Is she helping me to explore my own thoughts and feelings?

emotional well-being. Regardless of motivation, breaking the silence in a confidential and safe atmosphere is usually helpful.

If she is convinced that neither society nor her family can provide support, a woman may resist sharing her pregnancy and abortion even in the sanctity of a counselor's office. Whether a psychotherapist is emotionally removed or deeply engaged, a woman often fears she is being secretly judged. She may worry that the therapist will not be accepting of her "controversial" situation and could further contribute to her pain.

There are many psychotherapists who are truly non-judgmental and whose goal it is to support the personal growth and well-being of their patients. Psychological research has shown us that nonjudgmental pre- and post-abortion counseling can help women feel less isolated, mourn their chosen loss and place the event of their abortion in the overall context of their lives. Unfortunately, there can be a risk in receiving psychotherapeutic help when the therapist is biased.

> The family's survival depends on the shared sensibility of its members.
>
> —Elizabeth Stone
> *Black Sheep and*
> *Kissing Cousins*

Inappropriate counseling can increase post-abortion trauma. Several women confided that when they received psychotherapeutic help after their abortion, their emotional tension noticeably increased if their counselors attempted to impose their own dogmatic beliefs. These women felt that they had been subject to a negligent disregard for their personal values, unique lives and specific needs.

Nancy Adler, a psychological researcher from the University of California at San Francisco, has found that women whose "religion prohibits abortions and those who attend church more frequently" are more likely to have negative abortion responses. The religious bias against abortion may be reflected in conservative religious counselors as well.

Cynthia quit a conservative religious therapy group after attending only one session. She told us,

My priest gave me a referral to a church group for women who had
had abortions. He told me they would be compassionate. I went. It
was awful. I already felt loss, but I didn't think it helped me to be told
that I had committed a sin and that the fetus was a person I had
killed. I ended up quitting the group, but I also needed to call my
priest and tell him what had happened. I don't think he was prepared
to hear the harm that one hour of group therapy had done to me.
Thankfully, he encouraged me to find another group
through a community clinic.

> The family—that
> dear octopus from
> whose tentacles we
> never quite escape,
> nor, in our inmost
> hearts, ever quite
> wish to.
>
> —Dodie Smith
> *Dear Octopus*

Confused about where to safely turn for guidance,
afraid of the emotional risks inherent in seeking support, or certain that their pain will simply diminish over
time, women usually reject the possibility of professional
counseling. Professional help can be very useful, however,
when it is nonbiased and supportive.

Exercise Four:

1. Did you feel you needed any counseling at the time of your pregnancy or
   abortion? If so, did you seek it?
2. Was any counseling offered to you through a clinic or physician's office, or
   through a church, temple or community group?
3. If you received counseling, how did it affect your experience? How was it
   helpful? How was it unhelpful?
4. If you did not seek counseling, how did you make that decision?

Sharing with Friends and Family

There may be a risk when you turn to friends or loved ones for
support, as you cannot always predict what you will receive. You may
be reaching out for comfort, but you may receive condemnation and
confusion instead. No matter how much support you do or don't find,

your abortion decision with all its variations of emotional coloring, is one with which you alone must ultimately contend.

Women who confide in others try to choose carefully from among the friends who they believe will be supportive of their soul-searching or post-abortion discomfort. Sometimes they request support from someone they hope can provide it, but are disappointed—and sometimes their expectations are surpassed.

Cloe believed she made a good decision in whom to tell and not to tell. At the age of nineteen, she decided to withhold the news from the emotionally volatile boyfriend who had impregnated her, feeling that he would be unable to understand the complexity of her decision and, therefore, couldn't lend support. Instead, Cloe turned to two female friends who gave her comfort, and to her father, with whom she had a close relationship:

> I felt it shelter to speak to you.
> —Emily Dickinson
> Letter

I called my father and invited him to dinner. I decided to tell him. He handled it really well and asked if I needed any help. He was supportive and left me alone in terms of my decision making, never telling me what I should or shouldn't do.

Cloe felt thankful that she had two trusted friends and a helpful father, and that she did not have to go through the experience alone.

Many women successfully confide in their lovers or husbands. As a result, their sense of isolation is lessened, although they still feel a natural and predictable separateness, even from those most intimately involved in their dilemma. Meryl told us,

My boyfriend talked about it with me. He said he would come with me, he would do anything, whatever was best. He always said, "I trust that you have the best knowledge and the best access to information, and that you know what you're doing. I know what you're going through." I thought, "No, you really don't know." But he was simply trying to be nice and supportive in saying that and leaving the decision and planning up to me.

At other times, women's pain and aloneness are heightened when they break their silence to partners or family members who are unwilling or unable to lend support.

Lucy was only sixteen when she was date-raped by her sixteen-year-old boyfriend, Gary. The conception itself was traumatic, as was the moment she broke her silence and told him that she planned to abort. Already feeling isolated and without supportive friends or family to turn to, Lucy risked confiding in Gary. "Oddly enough," Lucy says, "he was the one person I felt closest to at the time." Although he voiced great concern for the five-week-old fetus, he refused to understand Lucy's emotional rape trauma or to support her desire to terminate the pregnancy. Lucy tells us,

> We want people to feel with us more than to act for us.
> —George Eliot
> Letter

> I wish I hadn't told him that I was pregnant. He absolutely didn't want to marry me, but he really wanted a baby. We talked and talked, and I cried. I begged him to explain his contradiction, but he couldn't or wouldn't. I'm not sure. He pressured me right to the end.

When Lucy made the decision to go ahead with her abortion, Gary called her mother, who rushed to the clinic intending to stop the procedure. A priest whom Lucy had met earlier at the clinic, and with whom she shared her fears and reasons for termination, met her mother in the lobby. He helped intercede for Lucy, calmly explaining why, at sixteen years of age, Lucy felt unprepared to parent a child. Now, with ten years of hindsight, Lucy believes that the priest she hardly knew was the only person in her life who sincerely cared about helping her. He was the least emotionally reactive and surprisingly had no other agenda aside from offering her emotional support.

Shanda, now thirty-eight years old, did not believe that she could find support within her family at the time of her pregnancy and wasn't sure which of her friends she could lean on when she had her abortion in 1983.

I decided to talk about myself in the third person. I told three of my friends that I'd heard of a girl at another school who was pregnant and that she was scared. When my friend Yolanda responded very compassionately, I knew she would be the person to ask for help. It was a good choice—she was really there for me. The clinic was $69 if you were pregnant and $39 if you wanted a suction extraction but showed negative on the pregnancy test. I had to bring a urine sample with me, so Yolanda gave me hers. She peed in a bottle at home before she met me at five o'clock that morning. In those days the difference of $30 meant eating for the week.

> Each friend represents a world in us, a world possibly not born until they arrive, and it is only by this meeting that a new world is born.
>
> —Anaïs Nin

Shanda's instincts were good in finding the right person to help, support and understand her specific needs.

Diane and her husband, Henry, already parents, grappled with a very different kind of conflict when faced with an unplanned pregnancy. After she discovered she was pregnant, Diane's first impulse was to have a third child. Although Henry was able to hear Diane's feelings and relate his own, any support he offered was marred by conflicts he was having in their marriage, problems he became aware of only after being confronted by the prospect of adding another child to their family.

Whereas Diane wanted unconditional support for her pregnancy, Henry could offer his full support only for healing their relationship. Diane confided that she became aware that an abortion, although not desired, was inevitable to serve the greater good of their marriage and their family. Both Diane and Henry told us that a thorough airing of their feelings, needs and desires helped them through the decision and abortion together.

Fifteen years later, pangs from that abortion infrequently surface. Diane is consoled about her loss in that the pregnancy forced the couple to look at their problems directly. Henry believes the painfully chosen loss saved their marriage and kept their family intact. Sharing their opposing needs was safe and helpful for each of them. Their predicament called for consensus, and their already established conflict-resolution skills supported the process of deciding what to do.

> Family life! The United Nations is child's play compared to the tugs and splits and need to understand and forgive in any family.
>
> —May Sarton
> *Kinds of Love*

Exercise Five:

1. Did you share the news of your pregnancy and abortion with friends or a significant other?
2. Whom did you choose to confide in and why?
3. Did you choose to keep this information private? Why?
4. Since the time of your abortion have you confided in others?
5. How has confiding in others, or deciding not to, helped or hurt you?

Loss of Privacy During the Abortion

No matter what lengths you may have gone to in order to secure and protect your own privacy, your pregnancy became "public" the moment you entered the medical community. When you disclosed the issue to doctors and strangers you abdicated your right to privacy—you had no choice.

Many times, a woman finds herself uncomfortable discussing the reasons why she chose to terminate a pregnancy, even with a doctor. This may be true even when the doctor is a woman's private physician with whom she has had a long, established relationship. Susan relates,

I felt that my relationship with a married man was a very private thing. That was the reason I couldn't have the baby. My personal doctor wanted a reason from me, but no reason was good enough for him. I finally told him the father was married. I felt like I had given up my privacy in telling him. What was worse is that the doctor didn't feel like this was a good enough reason for him! He wasn't happy about giving me the referral.

Susan's previously private life suddenly became public knowledge, and external judgments came her way—her greatest fear!

For a woman who has had multiple abortions, the anxiety of disclosing this information to medical professionals can elicit an even more pronounced fear of judgment. Wendy had told her long-standing family doctor about one abortion she'd had at a clinic, but could never imagine disclosing the full truth—that she had had three abortions. When Wendy joined an HMO and revealed her complete medical history to a new physician, her fears were realized:

> Cocooning: The need to protect oneself from the harsh, unpredictable realities of the outside world.
>
> —Faith Popcorn
> *The Popcorn Report*

I had an initial visit for a strep throat, but because it was my first visit, I had to fill out a complete medical history. I went in five months later because my period was late, and the doctor ran a pregnancy test without my approval. I instantly took that as being judged based on a previous situation.

Although many women do not share Susan's and Wendy's experiences, it comes as no surprise that nearly all the women with whom we spoke, even those who could afford to use the services of their personal physician, wanted to have their abortions at a clinic. They hoped that "going public" with medical personnel they had never met and would never encounter again might preserve a sense of privacy. They wanted to arrive and leave the clinic anonymously.

The self-protective anonymity women seek may, however, reinforce a sense of worthlessness. Sometimes, women feel like just another number, just another appointment in a busy day. Other times, they feel exposed by being required to disclose information that they would have preferred to keep secret.

Women tell us,

> Nothing's as good as holding on to safety.
>
> —Euripides
> *The Phoenician Women*

"It was called an 'anonymous abortion,' but it wasn't really anonymous. I had to give my social security number."

"I didn't want it written anywhere, ever, that I'd had an abortion. I gave a fake name."

"I felt a terrible loss of privacy when I was lined up with the other women like cattle."

"Wednesday was Abortion Day at the hospital. Ten gurneys and nine of us were there for an abortion. It was like an assembly line. Anyone would know why we were there."

Privacy was of the utmost importance to Meryl. Although she was surrounded by a broad network of friends and close family members, she chose to share the news of her pregnancy and abortion only with her fiancé and one girlfriend. Meryl's reasons for choosing as much privacy as possible included:

> I had neglected to use birth control, at the age of thirty, and felt a lot of shame. All my friends were having babies, and I didn't want any pressure to have one. I felt very depressed that, given three more years, I would be ready for this child—but I wasn't then.

Meryl decided that going to her private gynecologist was too emotionally risky for her at the time:

> He has a picture of his four children on his desk, and just about every woman who comes in there is pregnant. I would have felt

too awkward. When I go in for my yearly exam I will tell him, but I feel that I will be divulging something that will be perceived as negative.

To keep her abortion private from her doctor, Meryl decided to be part of a university study for the "morning-after pill." For Meryl, the experience was positive:

> The doctor was younger than me, very nice, and had a really wonderful bedside manner. When he walked into the room I thought, "Wow, this is different. This is good!" The nurses were six wonderful women. The only actual RN in the group was this feisty, tiny little Cuban woman named Anita, who was hilarious. She had me laughing and she was so nice. They were great, all of them.
>
> I did this on my own and with a sense of control. I found the program and drove to the hospital by myself. I'm glad I went through it this way. I'm not sure it was any less physically traumatic than a vacuum abortion, but emotionally it was right. I felt a sense of privacy, but I didn't feel alone.

Nothing is so burdensome as a secret.

—French proverb

Meryl was fortunate because her privacy strategy worked. She also had the unexpected benefit of a nonjudgmental staff who supported her.

Exercise Six:

1. Did you worry that you would be judged by medical professionals on your abortion day?
2. How might you have felt a loss of privacy?
3. How were you treated by professionals during your abortion procedure and afterward?

4. Did you feel respected or judged by nurses, a doctor or any clinical staff members?

Ongoing Feelings of Separation and Isolation

A woman's experience of separateness does not always end after her pregnancy has been terminated. The experience may remain part of her life history that she elects to keep private. She might later choose to share it with a physician, a future mate or a close friend, but rarely will she freely divulge the story of her abortion.

> Sometimes you just gotta trust that your secret's been kept long enough.
> —Anne Cameron
> *Daughters of Copper Woman*

Many women are at peace in their private memories. But others live without resolve if they remain unaware of the source of a chronic anxiety, the reasons for their decision to abort and the impact of their action on their lives in the future.

When we asked women, "Whom have you told about your pregnancy and abortion?" they usually stated that, aside from those in whom they confided at the time, they had told few or no others since. Their decision to maintain their privacy was often a reaction to the same stressor they faced during their original experience: they could not know whether they would be judged. At the same time, nearly all

Important Reasons for Reaching Out to Others

1. You don't feel alone.
2. You feel more connected to yourself when speaking to another.
3. You get emotional support.
4. Speaking aloud can clarify your thinking.
5. Sharing a secret with at least one person lightens a burden.
6. Sharing can soothe your pain and help you understand your reasons for the abortion.
7. You have someone to call for encouragement.

the women we spoke with believed that opting for total silence, especially when it led to depressing isolation, would not be a healthy choice.

Exercise Seven:

If you have ongoing feelings of separation and isolation, it may be time to consider breaking your silence. You took that first step when you began this book by breaking your silence with yourself. Breaking your silence with others may feel like a huge risk, especially if you fear that you will be judged.

> The human animal needs a privacy seldom mentioned, freedom from intrusion. He needs a little privacy quite as much as he wants understanding or vitamins or exercise or praise.
>
> —Phyllis McGinley
> *The Province of the Heart*

If you have broken your silence with a trusted "other" already, you can contact that person and let them know that you are presently working through unresolved feelings about your abortion and you might want their support again.

You might be thinking, "Give me one good reason why I should take this step." It is an important question, and the answer is simple: Secrets, when they make a person feel isolated, are dangerous. They can create shame. They can lead to guilt. They can keep pain from healing.

A shared secret, when received with understanding, such as a simple and accepting nod or "I hear you," ends your isolation and gives you the knowledge that you are not alone.

Breaking your silence means choosing one other person in the world and letting her or him know about your experience. You might choose to tell a close girlfriend or your significant other. You might decide to tell a trusted family member.

If there is no one in your immediate circle of friends or family whom you would trust, you can always turn to a professional counselor with whom you know your secret will remain confidential. Organizations such as Planned Parenthood are a good source for referrals to nonjudgmental counselors.

Take your time in finding the right person; it will be worthwhile.

When questioned further as to why they recoil from others' judgments, women answer: "It's no one's business," or "It was so long ago," or, most often, "I feel too much guilt." Because guilt occurs so frequently for post-abortion women, the next chapter examines this crucial and uncomfortable emotion and its implications in recovery.

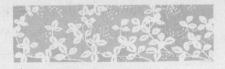

Chapter Four

Guilt

"I'm not afraid of storms, for I am learning how to sail my ship."
—Louisa May Alcott
Little Women

One would be hard pressed to find a post-abortion woman who has not felt some degree of guilt. It is normal. But, if you are a woman who has remained guilt ridden for a long time, the pain surrounding your abortion needs your attention.

If you feel guilty about a past abortion, it is necessary to understand what guilt is and its possible sources in order to find peace. In this chapter we will look at the definition of guilt and how it can be influenced by your family and the surrounding culture. Because women are usually attuned to other people's feelings, we will explore how this sensitivity toward relatedness may be disrupted by an abortion, setting in motion feelings of guilt. We will also look at guilt as a constructive post-abortion emotion which, when attended to with deep personal compassion, can even alert a woman to other areas in her life that are hurting her.

It is healthy to question yourself, because having an abortion was a significant decision. If your understanding remains incomplete, it is possible that there are feelings of guilt that you have not addressed.

Exercise One:

Answer the following questions. Write as much as you can in your journal for each answer:

> There's a period of life when we swallow a knowledge of ourselves and it becomes either good or sour inside.
>
> —Pearl Bailey
> *The Raw Pearl*

1. What does terminating a fetus mean to you?
2. How does having an abortion fit with your self-image?
3. Have you let yourself down?
4. Have you let the fetus down?
5. What parts of your inner life or soul may need tending?
6. How will you use the freedom from this childbirth to further your goals?
7. How have you used that freedom thus far?

Understanding the definition and the development of guilt as a normal human emotion is a step toward tracing the roots of the pain you might be living with now.

What Is Guilt?

In the most simple terms, guilt is the feeling that says: "I made a mistake." It is a response a child learns early in life—even before the age of five—from parents who tell her the "don'ts," "nos" and "shoulds" of behavior: "Don't jump on the bed," "No, you can't kick the cat," or "You should have kissed Aunt Bessie at the picnic."

During her early years, a little girl depends on parents and authority figures for validation in order to solidify her positive self-image. When she does something that doesn't meet with their approval, she responds by saying "I'm sorry." If she receives their forgiveness and secures their love and esteem once more, she feels better about herself. If she doesn't apologize, they may withhold their approval, which induces intolerable guilt. In order to stop awful feelings of guilt, the child relents and apologizes, accepting that it is better to give up what she wants to do than feel guilt for doing it.

At around five years of age a child becomes faced with a developmental challenge: she must learn to preserve some parental ideas that are truly constructive for her, while learning to let go of those messages that are contrary to her genuine "inner drummer." As she carves out her own identity, she begins to discover that she is different from Mom and Dad. She has her own opinions, emotions, temperament, likes and dislikes; for example, she may not like the doll her parents give her, but wants instead to play with her brother's baseball.

> Guilt is a rope that wears thin.
>
> —Ayn Rand
> *Atlas Shrugged*

With the exploration of her own special identity, feelings of anxiety and guilt naturally begin to arise in her. They are rooted in the fear that she might lose the love of those most important to her by risking their approval. But, if she has the encouragement of the adults in her life to pursue her real interests, the result will be positive self-esteem. In this way, guilt feelings are naturally mastered, and the child grows into a healthy independent thinker—or what psychotherapists call a "differentiated" person.

A girl who successfully tackles this stage of growth and initiates her own unique ideas without succumbing to paralyzing guilt learns a lesson that carries her into healthy adulthood: she does not have to adopt all of her parents' beliefs nor copy all of their behaviors—she can reject those that don't suit her.

Parents who encourage uniqueness and individuality in their children create future adults with self-esteem, the ability to manage personal guilt, and the skills necessary to make decisions that are in their own best interests regardless of the opinions of others.

Exercise Two:

If you are struggling with guilt feelings as an adult or have difficulty making decisions because you worry about how others will judge you, it is very important to look back at your childhood roots for healing. Think and write about the following:

> Children need models rather than critics.
>
> —Joseph Joubert
> *Pensees*

1. Did your parents encourage you to make some of your own decisions as a child?
2. Were you praised or punished when you listened to your "inner drummer"? How?
3. Were you afraid to make decisions that your parents might disagree with? Why or why not?
4. What were the lessons you learned about right and wrong behavior?
5. Do you struggle when making decisions as an adult?
6. Think back to a time in your childhood when you made a mistake that you were punished for. Did your parents use that mistake as an opportunity to teach you a lesson about right and wrong in a loving way?

Mature Guilt

If you are a woman who possesses a good sense of yourself, mature guilt functions as a "check system." When normal guilt feelings occur, you recognize that a part of your psyche sometimes acts like a child who is forced to live by other people's rules. At the same time, you know that you are a grown woman with your own belief system and values. You remind yourself that the process of living is never an absolute arrival, but a continuous uncovering of self-understanding that may require feeling normal guilt. As a differentiated adult, the normal guilt you experience over an action you have taken becomes a signal beckoning you to explore your present motivations and feelings about your choice: it is a message to "check" things out within yourself. You may discover you need a shift in your personal beliefs, or you may use the opportunity to reaffirm your values. As author Gail Sheehy maintains, during the experience of normal guilt, "buried parts of ourselves will demand incorporation or at least that we make the effort of seeing and discarding them."

Toxic Guilt

If you are a woman who does not possess a strong sense of yourself, challenging situations that occur in adulthood, like the resolution of an unwanted pregnancy, can create enormous internal anxiety, tension and toxic guilt. You might feel like a little child wondering, "Would Mom and Dad be mad at me if they knew I had an abortion?" You may feel unable to trust your own instincts and yearn to find out how others want you to behave in order to gain a sense of emotional well-being. Such thoughts signal that your guilt feelings need attention.

That most sensitive, most delicate of instruments— the mind of the child!

—Henry Handel Richardson
The Fortunes of Richard Mahoney: Ultima Thule

Mature Guilt

- is a check system
- sparks insight and reflection
- can cause you to transform old beliefs
- helps you know what is right for you

Toxic Guilt

- creates anxiety and tension
- makes you worry about what others will think about your choices and actions
- makes you give up what is right for you

Exercise Three:

1. In what ways might you feel guilty over your choice to terminate your pregnancy?
2. Have you been judged by others or feared that they would judge you if they knew about your abortion?
3. Who do you feel has judged your action? Who have you feared might judge you if you told them?

> A torn jacket is soon mended; but harsh words bruise the heart of a child.
> —Henry Wadsworth Longfellow
> "Table-Talk"
> *Driftwood*

The seeds of adult self-esteem, including both mature guilt and toxic guilt, are rooted in the family system.

The Family and Abortion Guilt

Family psychotherapist and educator Michael Frank describes the family as the major environment in which we become who we are, and "who we are is the basis from which we act." This means that a woman who finds herself with an unwanted pregnancy is aware of her family's beliefs and how her family members would react to this information, and also how her family would want her to respond.

Lisa was raised by her father after her parents divorced when she was eleven years old. Although she was twenty-six and living on her own when she became pregnant, Lisa had strong feelings of guilt when she imagined her father's reaction to her abortion. Lisa tells us,

> At the time I don't remember feeling guilt for myself that I was having an abortion. But when I thought of my father, I did feel guilt. I also felt terror that my father would hate me if he knew I'd broken a family rule: "You don't get pregnant out of wedlock and you don't have abortions!"

Although Lisa feared that her father would disapprove of her because of the crisis she faced, she was able to emotionally support herself. She had completed her education, established her career and developed a network of close friends. These accomplishments became a source of self-esteem for Lisa, and she felt she could trust her own self-judgment without relying on the approval of her father. Lisa says,

> My pregnancy and abortion were only one small part of me—one aspect of my overall character. My father would have confused it with my entire being. It's for the best that I didn't tell him. The fortunate irony is that he is the one who taught me to think for myself.

> If the child got shamed for feeling angry, sad or sexual, he will shame himself each time he feels angry, sad or sexual.
>
> —John Bradshaw
> Bradshaw on: The Family

Chris was only fourteen when she became pregnant and, unlike Lisa, had not mastered tolerating guilt. Chris was not yet mature enough to be emotionally self-supporting. She was living with her mother, who she knew would never approve of her sexual behavior nor be sympathetic to her pregnancy. Having internalized her mother's belief system, and still too young to have solidified her own values, Chris had "huge feelings of guilt and shame." She decided to keep silent about her abortion, but a short time later, her guilt erupted as defiance against her mother. In retrospect, Chris explains,

> I had a lot of growing up to do. I was wasting my time rebelling against my mom. Finally, when I was in college and far away from home, I realized I was still doing things to piss my mother off—only she didn't even know. It occurred to me, at that point, that I was protesting against myself for incidents that I felt guilty about: getting pregnant, having an abortion and letting myself down.

Chris's junior year in college was a turning point in her process of overcoming programmed guilt. She began initiating actions and behaviors to become her own person. She started to recognize that her feelings were all her own and that she must heal them for herself—not for her mother.

Even women who view their families as having been supportive often hesitate to discuss their abortion if they suspect their news might destroy the picture of their "perfect family," where anything and everything can be shared. Psychotherapist Michael Frank notes that guilt may arise when the "child" part of a woman begins to reason,

> What families have in common the world around is that they are the place where people learn who they are and how to be that way.
>
> —Jean Illsley Clarke
> *Self-Esteem: A Family Affair*

"My parents have been open to everything so far, so I don't want to push it because I couldn't stand the thought of them saying, 'No, this is it. This is one thing we can't accept.'" Because of this, girls and women usually decide whom to confide in depending upon the degree of support they anticipate receiving.

Cloe was twenty-three years old when she became pregnant. She shared the news with her father, whom she knew would be understanding, but did not confide in her mother despite Cloe's conviction that they were close. Twenty years later, she reflects,

I felt that my mother would be critical of me, and I didn't want to hear what she'd have to say. I think it goes back to my own unconscious shame. In reality, what would she have done? Put me down? Probably not. Was she going to lock me up in the house and tell me I couldn't have sex again in my life? In reality, she probably wouldn't have dissuaded me from having an abortion, as she is much more aware than that. But I felt real guilt that I made the mistake of getting pregnant.

The "secret" Cloe kept from her mother raised important questions for her: "Exactly what is okay to disclose in my family?" "Who do they want me to be?" and, ultimately, "What do I independently believe?" All of these are helpful questions to ask when long-term guilt is the consequence of a lack of self-examination.

Daisy originally insisted that guilt was never a part of her abortion experience. At the same time she didn't tell anyone in her family about her abortion. Daisy saw her certainty about having an abortion as proof that she lacked guilt. Some years later she came to realize that she could have certainty about her choice and feel normal guilt at the same time:

> I felt guilt in the sense that if my father had found out, he probably would have had a heart attack and died. Especially because he thought I was a virgin! He always put me on a pedestal. I had to get great grades, run for school offices, be really nice to my sisters. He couldn't have imagined I'd have sex or that I wasn't perfect. To have to deal with that bullshit really scared me more than anything about the whole situation.

> Healthy families are our greatest national resource.
> —Dolores Curran
> *Traits of a Healthy Family*

Fear of Confronting the Inner "Critic"

Fear is the primary emotion that keeps a woman from transforming her abortion pain. Fear can bind her to a false self-image. She fears that she will feel regret, anger, guilt and confusion or hear internalized voices of wrongdoing. She fears that she may be shattered if she explores the meaning of her abortion. Rather than opening a can of worms, she opts to linger in denial of her pain.

Some women fear that they do not deserve healing. They suspect that their action to abort was so ethically, morally or spiritually questionable that they deserve no relief. Either side of the coin produces the same result—an emotionally stunted woman walking through her years on earth wearing a mask designed by her parents and society, which she herself cannot see through.

Transformation requires that a woman no longer be a victim to her inner "critic." In this pursuit she must let go of her rigid and naive concept that life is supposed to be easy and never requires tough calls.

Only a woman who is willing to face her fear of what her "critic" is telling her, and discover and live by her true values, can move into her authentic self.

Daisy's concerns about her father helped identify guilt feelings stemming from her failure to be a "superwoman." At first, she saw this only in relation to her father, but then she realized that she couldn't be a superwoman to herself either. Her guilt feelings helped lead her to recognize herself in a less perfectionistic light; she acknowledged that she was not perfect. She reaffirmed the importance of her life goals, which included having children at a later time, and accepted that she had made sacrifices to reach them.

> The family the soul wants is a felt network of relationships, an evocation of a certain kind of interconnection that grounds, roots, and nestles.
>
> —Thomas Moore
> *Soul Mates*

If you are a woman who is unaware of the psychological forces that drive your life, you may be a sitting duck for inner critical voices. Responding as a young child would, you are apt to feel like a "bad girl" who has disobeyed an authority greater than herself. If you realize that you are inflicting this punishment upon yourself, you can choose to explore your inner life and trace the sources of these programmed punitive voices. The guilt you may feel from having an abortion can become a springboard into self-knowledge, leading you to realize that you have yet to fully separate from your parents and their values in order to stand on your own firm ground. Biological age does not always match emotional age, but doing inner work at any age is better than not doing it at all.

Exercise Four:

1. Did you have feelings of guilt about sharing or not sharing your abortion with your family?

2. If you shared it, did you feel support or were you punished for doing the "wrong thing"?

3. If you chose to keep your pregnancy and abortion a secret, did you fear that you would be seen as wrong or less than perfect, or that you would risk losing your family's love and respect? Do you feel this now?

The Culture's Effects on Guilt

In addition to the influence of your family, the culture you live in can have a powerful impact on your beliefs, self-image and emotions. Like your childhood family, the culture offers its own beliefs about "right" and "wrong" behaviors and can elicit feelings of guilt, conflict and remorse.

As a girl matures into adulthood she must reconcile what she was taught at home with information presented by teachers, friends, the media and organizations to which she belongs. By consciously weighing the barrage of conflicting views against her own values, she begins to see herself both as a member of society and as someone who has her own identity. Ideally, she sorts through all of these new views and accepts those that she genuinely believes are valid, while disregarding the rest. It is a more sophisticated version of the psychological task she faced in her family beginning at the age of five.

> I seem to have an awful lot of people inside me.
>
> —Edith Evans

Just as a woman learns that there are members of her family who may or may not accept her abortion, she discovers that society has its own array of voices. While some of these voices may foster personal development, others may inflict debilitating judgments. Anne tells us,

I felt so loved by the people around me and so despised by strangers I didn't even know! It seemed like every time I turned on the news I was hearing another angry voice telling me that I, personally, was a bad human being for having an abortion. Even though I regard myself as pretty aware, those "other" voices kept telling me, "You are wrong. You are evil." Intellectually, I knew they were wrong to judge me, but just like me, these other folks felt so sure. I couldn't help but wonder, "Are they right?" I had to work hard to reaffirm my own truth and deal with the guilt.

Many women, like Anne, are keenly aware of the presence of outside "other voices" espousing contrary views on abortion. Some women hear those voices as mere background chatter, while others attend to them with caution and concern.

Exercise Five:

Use the following to ascertain the degree to which you may be unknowingly influenced by "other voices."

> Sexuality is the great field of battle between biology and society.
>
> —Nancy Friday
> *My Mother/My Self*

1. Take a moment and try to hear the "other voices" that might have spoken negative messages to you as you went through your abortion experience.
2. Are these voices still alive in your mind today?
3. Which cultural voices are you sensitive to today?
4. Make a thorough list of what these voices told you then, and what they may be telling you now, about your action and about women who have abortions.

A woman with a heightened sensitivity to the culture's mixed voices hears them everywhere: the sermon of a pastor, a conversation overheard in a coffee shop, the words of a newscaster, a headline in the morning paper, a discussion in a college class or a debate at a dinner party.

If a woman feels unresolved internal conflict over her decision to abort, the voices become even more effective in penetrating and sparking her guilt. Intellectually, she may be aware that her past action would not be met with unconditional approval by the entire world, and so she questions herself: "Have I done the right thing? Am I a good person?"

If a woman is conscious of her own belief system and has well-defined values, she is able to differentiate her true voice from the "other voices" in the culture. She can support her stance and manage any normal guilt feelings that might arise through a process of constructive self-investigation, which may expand or change her ever evolving identity.

The Culture and Sexual Guilt

Cultural messages include ethics, morals, religious beliefs, peer pressures, the media's input, heroic images, mythology and images of sexuality. Finding your way through the external onslaught to your own core beliefs is an arduous task, but cultural messages regarding sexuality are particularly powerful. They are a common source of guilt for many women, and a potential source of guilt for post-abortion women in particular.

A single male who follows his sexual drive is often hailed as a "manly man," while a sexually active single woman may be considered "promiscuous" or lacking in moral character. As a result, sex has become a frequent source of guilt for women. The truth is, if human beings (as "human animals") did not have a powerful sex drive, the species would die out. This is a law of nature. Nevertheless, a woman may mercilessly berate herself for enjoying a short hour of passion.

> A sex symbol becomes a thing. . . . I just hate to be a thing.
>
> —Marilyn Monroe
> Quoted in Ms. magazine

A woman who feels conflicted over responding to her sexual desires and subsequently finds herself with an unplanned pregnancy may experience a torrent of guilt. She will likely dismiss any rational voices and fixate on those voices that corroborate her shame: "I'm a woman with questionable morals for having sexual urges, and if I hadn't acted on those base urges, I wouldn't be pregnant now."

When a woman, even one who is not conflicted over her sexual nature, terminates an unwanted pregnancy, she inevitably hears the judgments of society ringing in her ears. She knows, as author and psychotherapist Angela Bonavoglia tells us, that the myriad judgments put upon women for choosing to abort a fetus "provide ample evidence that a society's attitudes toward abortion cannot be separated from that society's attitudes toward sexuality, particularly female sexuality." How a woman responds to the culture's monstrous guilt complex, which dictates that she "should" feel guilt because her "promiscuity" led her to the controversial abortion, depends upon her self-esteem and insight.

Young women, vulnerable to their own conflicting emotions over their natural sexual urges, are especially disarmed by society's messages. Advertising, television and movies are brimming with images of scantily clad young women presented as desirable females. Yet if young women dress and act in accordance with these images, they are considered too sexually overt. Trapped in a cultural paradox, they may want to be recognized as being desirable, but fear being seen as "sluts" for having sexual feelings. These young women will almost certainly punish themselves with guilt if they become pregnant—"After all," their critical inner voices tell them, "you should have known better!"

> Females are naturally libidinous, incite the males to copulation, and cry out during the act of coition.
>
> —Aristotle
> *Historia animalium*

Conflicting cultural messages are particularly harmful to a woman who has been faced with an unwanted pregnancy because of a rape. Anita, forty years old, relates the following story:

> I was date-raped this year by a man whom I had just started seeing and really liked. I was wracked with guilt trying to figure out how I had created the situation: Was I too suggestive? Did I wear the wrong clothes? It was all the stereotypical guilt stuff. I didn't even report it to the police because I was so sure that they would see me as the "bad guy." It wasn't only that I had seen too many movies of the woman being blamed. It was because I knew too many true stories of her really being condemned, and I couldn't stand the thought of working through that stuff publicly.

When Anita discovered that she was pregnant, her guilt took on even greater proportions. She lied to her doctor about the circumstances of her pregnancy, never confided in a friend and only disclosed the truth of her experience in our interview.

Women who are raped and those who find themselves pregnant through incest often feel unaccountably guilt ridden. They frequently remain secretive and filled with remorse, fearing that, should the truth of their experience be known, others will wonder, "Did she lead him on?" "Did she enjoy it?" "Could she have prevented it?" Their work is to pose the questions to themselves and answer them from a compassionate inner place rather than from imagined external judgments. These women's healing work also includes the trauma of the rape. (See the Resources list in the appendix for rape and incest recovery sources.)

The use or misuse of birth control, when conception has taken place, also haunts women. They reveal a consistent belief, highly conditioned by the culture, that birth control is ultimately the woman's responsibility.

Vicky, who hadn't used birth control, candidly explained the emotional pain she felt as a young woman trying to suppress her sexual desires in order to comply with the culture's restrictive view on female sexuality and her church's edict for celibacy before marriage. Unexpectedly, she elected to defy both culture and church:

> If you haven't forgiven yourself something, how can you forgive others?
>
> —Dolores Huerta
> "Stopping Traffic: One Woman's Curse"
> *The Progressive*,
> Barbara L. Baer

Twenty years ago sex was a sin, sex was evil; even just contemplating it was committing this horrendous act. So I didn't plan on having sex and so never even considered birth control. I was young when I met Robert. He was Catholic like I was. We were necking and, in a moment of passion, we started making love. I had been taught about the rhythm method, and I knew I wasn't ovulating by the math I had done in my head. Obviously my body was counting differently from how I was, and I got pregnant. The guilt was enormous, and I think it is still with me today. How could I have let myself get so carried away? The doctor who confirmed my pregnancy was direct and instructive. He said, "Rhythm is for musicians and dancers."

Marla also identified with sexually based guilt when her birth control failed. She says,

> I got pregnant last year, when I was thirty-five, and immediately felt really stupid. Here I was, educated and knowing all about how to use birth control. I had been one of those women who always preached that abortion was not a means of birth control and women who used it that way were reckless. I mean, hasn't that been a popular credo? So, when my diaphragm failed to work, I imagined a million people shaking their fists in my face and preaching away. The irony is that I had unprotected sex in the past, never got pregnant and never felt any guilt.

> Truth is the only safe ground to stand upon.
> —Elizabeth Cady Stanton
> *The Woman's Bible*

Sara, too, saw her sexuality as a contributor to her feelings of guilt. She shares,

> I felt responsible because I chose not to use birth control. I didn't even want my boyfriend to get up and get a condom. Then I had to pay for it. I was upset with myself because for those couple of minutes of sex, look what I've had to go through.

Vicky, Marla, Sara and countless other women like them have suffered from the implied moral code dictating female sexual behavior that is woven into the very fabric of culture. Rather than treating themselves with reason and compassion, they have punished themselves for making a "mistake" that they believe they could have prevented. They believe they should have been able to take foolproof measures to prevent conception, especially if they initiated sexual intercourse.

However, women often fail to remember the objective facts of biological productivity and womanhood. With thirty to forty years of fertility in a woman's lifetime, possibly 520 ovulation cycles and a compelling human sex drive, an enormous number of pregnancies result—some wanted and others not. It is, therefore, no wonder that 46 out of 100 women in the United States experience an abortion in their lifetime. The pregnancy might be a result of the lack or misuse of birth control, birth control failure or simply youthful ignorance regarding sexual reproduction. Such an awareness reminds women that unplanned pregnancy is not always a matter of reckless behavior, but simply a result of numerical odds.

Exercise Six:

1. What messages have you received from the culture about women and sexual behavior?

2. How have those messages influenced your self-image as a sexual woman?

3. Have you felt that your own misuse, neglect or choice of birth control led to your pregnancy and abortion?

4. If you became pregnant through a rape, incest, a one-night stand or a relationship that you felt was unhealthy, what messages do you believe society has cast or would cast upon you?

> A friend can tell you things you don't want to tell yourself.
> —Frances Ward Weller
> *Boat Song*

Acting against Relatedness

Often a woman's decision to terminate a fetus is in stark contrast to her drive toward relatedness. It is a drive that makes her seek connections with others and give to others, makes her hope that others will "like" her and tells her that she "should" want to protect others—including her fetus. This drive is essential to her identity as a woman and is recognized by society as distinctly female. When the drive is not felt or met, guilt may result.

Until recently, our understanding of the psychological growth of a human being was based primarily upon male thinking. Developmental theories were predominantly created by men, such as Lawrence Kohlberg, Jean Piaget and Erik Erikson, who largely employed males as their subjects. Many of these theorists espoused the view that the goal of psychological growth was emphatic self-reliance. A male went through childhood, teen years and adulthood striving to gain autonomy in his quest to become a whole, healthy individual who would rely on no one but himself.

While the notion that "all healthy human beings strive for a total sense of individuality" is a valuable one, many aspects of this theory have limited applications for contemporary women.

This is the sacred marriage of the feminine and masculine—when a woman can truly serve not only the needs of others but can value and be responsive to her own needs as well.

—Maureen Murdock
The Heroine's Journey

Women have long believed that relatedness is enriching and that a sense of self is developed through the experience of sharing. They have confided their deepest secrets to female friends and have felt a consistent urge to be known and to know others. Husbands and boyfriends often stand in amazed disbelief at the level of honesty and disclosure among women. In fact, when asked, "Who is your best friend?" most women name their closest female friend, while men usually name their wife or girlfriend. The intimacy these men have been so unable to experience with other men is, for so many women, commonplace. And the intimacy that is commonplace for women is exactly what can make terminating a fetus guilt provoking.

Today, women stand in the shoes of both male and female modes of personal development. They can become presidents of the school board or corporate officers with the same self-driven, autonomous panache that has characterized men. These women usually know that when they come up with a great idea or innovation, its meaning is not simply reflected in personal achievement or an increased profit margin, but also through its impact on other human beings.

Because of this compelling dual perspective, a woman may feel conflicted when deciding to terminate a fetus. She feels the tension between the typically male model of autonomy, which urges her to meet her own needs, and the female model of relatedness, which reminds her of the relationship between herself and the fetus in her womb.

Sometimes a woman's conscientious abortion decision is based upon a desire to keep her present life uninterrupted or upon her need to secure future goals. When women reflect on their reasons for terminating a pregnancy, they can see how these combined masculine and feminine models have influenced their choice. The student who chooses to abort meets her own needs by staying in school and completing her education, thereby refusing to take on adult responsibilities for which she feels unprepared. The mother-housewife who chooses to abort meets her needs by remaining available to the children she already has, to her spouse and to her vast commitments as a homemaker. The working mother who chooses to abort meets her own needs by ensuring that she does not become over-whelmed and can continue to meet the demands that already exist in her life, thus allowing herself to enjoy her job and her family at a continued level of responsibility. A childless career woman meets her needs by fostering her personal and professional life, knowing that she does not want to accommodate a child's schedule.

> One can never consent to creep when one feels an impulse to soar.
> —Helen Keller
> *The Story of My Life*

A woman may feel guilty or embarrassed to admit that self-direction (the traditionally male-oriented model emphasizing auton-omy) influenced her decision to abort. And sometimes no amount of logic will lessen her guilt when she recalls her past action. Lynette tells us,

> Physically and biologically it was wrong to abort. The life force wanted to come forward. But my husband was unemployed. And in my career, things looked like they might take off. A fourth baby would have taken me way off the track I'd worked so hard to get on. So, yes, I have regrets. I'll never know for sure what could have happened. I do know I like my work and my family as it is. This soothes my guilt.

Lynette, and other women like her, struggle with their guilt as they juggle the "autonomy" and "relatedness" ways of being a whole person. Despite their drive toward relatedness and the culturally embedded notion that women "should" always respond to nature's call to motherhood, they are choosing to nurture other priorities and have abortions. And, like Lynette, as responsible as they might have been when making their abortion decisions, some women later fear they may have been uncomfortably self-serving. This is neither abnormal nor unusual.

> I do not want to die . . . until I have faithfully made the most of my talent and cultivated the seed that was placed in me until the last small twig has grown.
>
> —Käthe Kollwitz
> *The Diaries and Letters of Käthe Kollwitz*

Female Emotional Development

In the last ten years, female psychologists such as Carol Gilligan have emerged with new theories and insights about how women develop. These new theories have turned a century of psychological models upside down. Although both the new and old models agree that the developmental goal of men and women is to become fully actualized, the major difference between them is that women are thought to achieve a sense of individuality largely through their interactions and intimate relationships with other people.

Women have shouted a resounding "Yes!" to these new theories. Interdependency and relatedness no longer imply stalled development, moral inferiority or "co-dependency." Instead, they are viewed as essential tools in the female journey toward wholeness. Author Emily Hancock believes this when she asks, "How is it that we have polarized the human agenda, lionizing separation and independence, leaving out entirely, meaningful connections between people and the human capacities for intimacy, empathy, care and compassion?" Author Jean Baker Miller agrees when she flatly states, "women stay with, build on, and develop in a context of attachment and affiliation with others."

Integrating these male and female models is a psychological balancing act for many women. Seldom are they totally identified with the sole achiever seeking autonomy at all costs, nor are they only identified with the "relatedness and the domestic caregiver" role. They are both.

Philosopher Paul Tillich has suggested that the greatest guilt comes not to the person who resists fulfilling others' needs, but to the person who does not fulfill her own destiny. Thus, a woman who does not sacrifice a pregnancy, and carries her fetus to term, may feel guilty for failing to nurture herself.

Jessica tells us,

I'd rather feel guilty for having an abortion than feel guilty for having a child I didn't want.

Here Jessica reveals that she takes mature responsibility for her abortion and that she is able to tolerate the normal guilt that accompanies it.

A woman may feel guilt for aborting a fetus and, in doing so, guilt for meeting her own needs. But, had she not chosen abortion, she might have been left with guilt for neglecting her destiny combined with guilt for poorly raising a child she didn't want.

If you are experiencing post-abortion guilt, self-examination can bring constructive results.

> I have been in Sorrow's kitchen and licked out all the pots. Then I have stood on the peaky mountain wrapped in rainbows, with a harp and a sword in my hands.
>
> —Zora Neale Hurston
> *Dust Tracks on a Road*

Exercise Seven:

1. Have you ever felt guilt for choosing your life plans over the potential life of the fetus you terminated?
2. How did having an abortion promote your independent growth?
3. How might you have let yourself down regarding your goals by having your abortion?

Making Guilt Constructive

A goal of adult individuals is to accept full responsibility and accountability for their actions. A post-abortion woman achieves this goal by accepting that her actions were deliberate and that she possesses a thorough understanding of why she chose to act as she did. Any guilt feelings she experiences can function constructively when they urge sincere self-examination rather than self-induced punishment.

Guilt can apply to transgressions committed against another person or against an overriding moral or social code. And guilt can also arise, even more painfully, from infractions against our essential core selves. Author Judith Viorst believes that the person who feels a true and mature guilt fears the anger of her own conscience and a loss of self-love, rather than her parents' anger and risking their love.

> The strongest principle of growth lies in human choice.
>
> —George Eliot
> *Daniel Deronda*

A mature post-abortion woman suffering from guilt may be most distressed over causing herself pain. She may feel guilt because she "messed up" her birth control or "foolishly" trusted her lover to "pull out" before orgasm, got pregnant and subsequently terminated a fetus despite any previous values and self-image to the contrary.

Several women we interviewed reported feeling surprised by their guilt reactions after their abortion. They stated that even though their choice would be the same had they to do it again, they found themselves struggling with the unexpected notion that they had inadvertently hurt themselves. They later felt guilty and critically judged what they once considered their best option.

If the termination of a fetus is unresolved, a woman's latent guilt and subsequent resolution may occasionally be triggered by other events. Melanie tells us,

> Two years after my abortion, my husband and I were watching a film on TV of a child being born. It was the first time I'd seen a birth from beginning to end—from the little peanut through the birth process. By the time it got to the end, both of us were sobbing. I asked him if it was because of the abortion. And he said, "Yes." It was very painful, yet it helped. We got the opportunity to let go together—even

though it was two years later. After that there was a sense of resolution. I accepted the fact of what I had done. I could bear it and mourn it.

Melanie and her husband turned what could have been subtle destructive guilt into constructive guilt by acknowledging their emotions and allowing themselves to grieve and share their feelings.

Women who have accepted their abortion with the aid of constructive guilt can recount times when this emotion urged them to understand their balance between autonomy and relatedness, to face the enormity of their decision to abort and to integrate that experience into the rest of their lives.

> Happy or unhappy, families are all mysterious.
>
> —Gloria Steinem
> *Outrageous Acts and Everyday Rebellions*

Regardless of the degree of guilt or regret, all the women we interviewed were grateful for the chance to relate their stories. Through the sharing came more healing.

Exercise Eight:

In order to transform destructive guilt into constructive guilt, you must respond to guilt feelings as a signal that there is inner work to accomplish, rather than as a command that you must feel bad about yourself. Guilt is a tool for inquiry, and you can begin by asking yourself the following questions:

1. What are you feeling guilty about?
2. How independent in your thinking were you when you got pregnant?
3. What were your reasons for having an abortion?
4. What did you sacrifice by having an abortion?
5. What did you gain?

Simply stating, "I had no other options," or "I was stupid to do what I did" will not quell any guilt feelings you may have unless you truly believe that at the time of your abortion no other options seemed as right as the decision to terminate. If, in your self-examination, you recognize there may have been another acceptable, albeit far less desirable, option, your healing work is to compassionately understand how you reached the abortion decision. Then you may face and mourn your limitations, possibly mourning the loss of the fetus, and in doing so broaden your self-view to include imperfections and vulnerability.

Because guilt is often accompanied by anger, we will now turn our attention to how abortion can evoke this powerful emotion in women.

Chapter Five
Anger

"I have a right to my anger, and I don't want anybody telling me I shouldn't be,
that it's not nice to be, and that something's wrong with me because I get angry."
—Maxine Waters
in *I Dream a World*
Brian Lanker

It is common for women to feel anger over the myriad complications
brought into their lives by an unplanned pregnancy. Identifying the
sources of your anger and resolving the discomfort it brings is an
essential step in post-abortion healing because anger, when left unhealed, can lead to ongoing emotional pain.

Anger, like guilt, carries energy that can be used positively or
negatively. When anger is recognized and expressed constructively, it
can be transformative. When it is denied and repressed, however, anger
can foster feelings of bitterness, victimization and depression.

It is necessary to recognize and specifically identify the anger you
may be carrying, in order to free it.

Transforming your anger may be necessary for both your psychological and physical health. Many medical doctors and psychotherapists

believe that repressed anger, and the stress it elicits, can manifest in physical symptoms such as colitis, ulcers, migraine headaches and stomach upset. When emotions are recognized, understood and resolved in positive ways, says author and psychoanalyst Marion Woodman, they do not have to get our attention through physical "dis-ease."

Exercise One:

Anger is something we feel. It exists for a reason and always deserves our respect and attention.
—Harriet Goldhor Lerner
The Dance of Anger

If you are feeling anger related to your abortion, consider the following in your journal:

1. Make a list of those things that angered you about your unwanted pregnancy.
2. Make a list of those things that angered you about your abortion.
3. How do you feel when you hear about friends', sisters' or other women's abortions?
4. How did you express your anger at the time of your pregnancy? And at the time of your abortion?
5. In general, how do you express anger now?
6. Do you easily anger?
7. Do you worry you feel anger too frequently? Could it be associated with abortion events?
8. Have you ever felt so angry that you suffered a headache or other physical symptoms?

This chapter will help you identify the sources of your post-abortion anger and find ways to constructively express that anger and transform it from a stifling emotion to a motivating force for change. Anger, as you will see, is a natural, necessary and multifaceted emotion that can play a key role in your abortion healing.

Outside forces form and shape how we handle anger on a daily basis. To understand post-abortion anger, it is necessary to decipher the messages you have received regarding anger from your early family and from society—especially messages regarding women's anger.

Messages from Family and Culture

Families often mismanage anger. As children, girls may have witnessed their parents' anger turn into terrifying rage. They may have experienced confusing passive–aggressive enactments of anger. Many girls have been erroneously taught that anger is an unacceptable emotion and been told to "Go to your room until you calm down." Or they may have experienced the complete denial of anger as if it did not exist at all. While

Perhaps You Have Felt Anger Because

- you neglected to use birth control;
- your birth control failed;
- your lover didn't "pull out" before orgasm;
- you were date-raped;
- you discovered that the baby you had planned for had a serious genetic defect;
- you felt you gave up a possible child and now wish you hadn't;
- you felt unsupported or judged by your doctor or clinic staff;
- you were criticized when you told someone about your unwanted pregnancy or abortion;
- you went through the experience alone;
- you have never told anyone about your abortion and feel like you are carrying a secret burden;
- your abortion was a financial hardship;
- your lover tried to make you carry the fetus to term;
- your lover was married and couldn't be involved;
- your lover was mad that you became pregnant;
- the pregnancy and abortion caused havoc in your family life;
- being a woman includes painful choices;
- your pregnancy pushed you into an unscheduled life passage;
- you felt forced to challenge your spiritual beliefs;
- your job or work suffered in some way.

> Let not the sun go down on your wrath.
> —Ephesians 4:26

little boys often play aggressive games, such as "soldiers" or "cops and robbers," wherein they freely express anger and act out death and dying, little girls most often play dolls and board games, wherein gentler emotions are sanctioned and cooperative nonviolent enactments are the norm. Because of these familial and societal distortions, women seldom learn to appropriately, comfortably or freely express their own anger.

Our feelings are our most genuine paths to knowledge.

—Audre Lorde,
Black Women Writers at Work, Claudia Tate, ed.

In therapy, adult women frequently relate examples of anger being mishandled in their childhood families. They initially state with pride, "When I was growing up no one in my family ever got angry, and I don't get angry either." Other women recount stories of violent outbursts, constant bickering or physical abuse. In response, they may have opted to either scream and yell like their parents or entirely suppress their own anger and never act mad. It is sad to hear women describe their childhood experiences, because the healthy truth is quite different from what they were conditioned to believe: anger is a natural emotion, everyone feels angry at one time or another, and it should be expressed in appropriate ways.

Compounding the psychological wounds inflicted upon all children in a family ill equipped to handle anger, daughters are most often raised—consciously or not—to squelch their expression of anger, according to researchers Kaplan and Bean. Schooled in this way, a female child is unable to validate an essential part of her emotional life or practice healthy ways in which to communicate normal feelings of aggression and hostility. As a young woman beginning a life independent from her family, she may believe that she has no right to express her anger, even if she wants to do so.

Standing upon this restrictive emotional foundation, a woman's angry silence is further reinforced by the culture she lives in. As Harriet Goldhor Lerner, author of The Dance of Anger, tells us, beginning in childhood the culture teaches girls that feminine women are absolutely devoid of anger and aggressiveness. These messages continue into adulthood, and "So strong are societal prohibitions against female anger, that the angry woman may be condemned, even if she is waging a bloodless and humane revolution for her own legitimate rights."

If she does express her anger, a woman may become the recipient of shaming cultural myths that tell her, "Men are assertive but women [who act that way] are bitchy," "Men are outspoken but women [who act that way] are pushy," and "Men are powerful but women [who act that way] are overbearing." If she lacks the internal strength and clarity to disarm these untruths, she may find herself living out the repressive lessons of her childhood: "Sugar and spice and everything nice, that's what little girls are made of."

> You can't change the music of your soul.
>
> —Katherine Hepburn
> *Esquire*

It is understandable why many women struggle to own and appreciate their authentic anger. And it is understandable why women who define themselves as "bad" for having legitimate anger hesitate before expressing their feelings or confronting the source of their emotional response. Instead, according to Lerner, they opt to feel "hurt" (a seemingly acceptable female emotion) in situations wherein anger is appropriate. Stuck in this emotional bind, their anger cannot be resolved because it is not recognized and named for the emotion that it is.

It is common to find a "hurt" post-abortion woman. Women tell us of feeling wounded, not simply because their experience was wounding—though it may have been—but because they do not believe themselves entitled to feel or express the anger connected to their abortion.

Exercise Two:

1. What are your earliest memories of anger in your home growing up?

2. Were you told not to be angry?

3. How were you taught to deal with anger as a child?

4. In what ways did other family members differ from you in their expressions of anger?

5. What sources outside your family influenced your feelings about anger? Consider teachers, the media, friends, etc.

6. What basic "rules" about anger did you take from your family into adulthood?

7. Who was the most accepting of your angry feelings in the past? Who is the most accepting now?

> Because society would rather we always wore a pretty face, women have been trained to cut off anger.
>
> —Nancy Friday

8. Who was the least accepting of any angry feelings you had in the past? Who is the least accepting now?

9. What did you feel angry about at the time of your abortion? Why?

10. At the time of your abortion, where was your anger directed? Why?

11. Did you feel anger at yourself? God? Your doctor?

12. Did you turn anger into "hurt"?

Feeling Shame about Feeling Anger

Post-abortion women face a special challenge when confronting their anger. Not only are they attempting to deal with an emotion they may feel uncomfortable approaching, but they are often reluctant to admit they are angry over an event they feel responsible for creating. If this is true for you, you may feel shame for feeling anger.

If you feel responsible for your unplanned pregnancy you may experience an internal resistance to exploring your anger. You may

Ways to Overcome Your Shame

- resist seeking safety in shame as a way to avoid your anger;
- accept that you are entitled to be angry;
- objectively examine your reasons for being angry with yourself, other people and the entire experience of your pregnancy and abortion.

believe that, because you "recklessly" became pregnant, you have "no right" to feel any anger and are filled with shame if you do. In your shame you may perceive the expression of anger to be a luxury you are not entitled to. And, from this place, you may punish yourself, saying, "If anyone or anything should be the target of my anger it is me, so I'll just shut up and suffer."

This is a double bind for a woman. If you realize that you have anger, it is important that you confront the emotion which you believe you have little entitlement to feel. If you resist feeling anger and resort to being a "hurt" woman, you may be trapped in ongoing misery and pain with no possibility for self-exploration, resolution or for-giveness.

The path out of this inner torture chamber requires that you commit yourself to addressing the reality of your anger. To remain hurt and ashamed may protect you from experiencing forbidden feelings, but it also serves to pro-long your distress.

> Feelings are the fine instruments which shape decision-making in an animal cursed and blessed with intelligence, and the freedom which is its corol-lary.
>
> —Willard Gaylin
> *Feelings: Our Vital Signs*

Exercise Three:

To confront and explore your anger may not be easy—anger can be a frightening and uncomfortable emotion. But if you want to secure a sense of well-being, you must be willing to endure self-examination and refute society's views of women and their right to anger. Your initial confrontation with your anger may be difficult, but the end result may be genuine self-knowledge and a lessening of your post-abortion pain.

1. In what ways might shame be related to your expression of anger?
2. How might you be caught in a double bind, or a lose-lose position, about exploring your anger?
3. In what ways is self-questioning difficult for you? Do you become dis-tracted? Do you focus on another person?
4. How are you feeling while writing in your journal at this very moment?

Integrating the Inner Mother

The struggle to come to grips with the forces that drive one's inner life is formidable. But if a woman can understand and integrate her inner aspects, she gains strength, which can help her to accept her decision to end a pregnancy. Integration also allows her to see the reasons for the anger she might experience and to view the expression of anger as essential to her well-being.

Although "nice ladies" are not very good at feeling angry, we may be great at feeling guilty.

—Harriet Goldhor Lerner

The Dance of Anger

Just as a woman has an "inner worker," "inner friend," or "inner child," she also has an "inner mother." The strength of the "inner mother" is manifest in various ways. Traditionally, the mother figure is experienced by women as the creator and sustainer of life, the first object of an infant's love, and the source that fills all early childhood needs.

The nurturing aspect of the inner mother is culturally reinforced. We are raised to believe, says author Nancy Friday, that "mother love is different from other kinds of love. It is not open to error, doubt or to the ambivalence of ordinary affections." Mother love, we are taught, is always life giving and never life destroying.

However, the "all-good" mother who conceives and sustains life is only one aspect of the inner mother. The true "inner mother" also has a driving force that creates endings as a natural part of living. It is a force that can be witnessed in mothers of all species. Female spiders may eat their mates to feed their young. Second-rank female wolves will destroy their pups to nurture the dominant female's litter. Mothers speak of their instinct to harm anyone who threatens their children. And, sometimes, women choose to destroy fetuses they feel unable to care for as, after an abortion, a woman's life-sustaining energies may be used to better care for herself or her present children.

The instinct, and often the conscious choice, to allow for endings is an integral part of female existence—a normal part of a woman's "inner mother." It is a truth that contradicts the revered image of the all-loving inner mother we cling to and, as females, strive to emulate whether we are personally mothers ourselves or not. It is a part of ourselves we cannot escape.

Through her choice to terminate a pregnancy, the post-abortion woman comes face-to-face with her abilities to create and destroy. If she has neither recognized nor honored the coexistence of these inner abilities, she may find herself in a psychological bind: having exercised her power to create an ending, she no longer fits the image of who she believes she "should" be.

> The ideal mother, like the ideal marriage, is a fiction.
> —Milton R. Sapirstein
> *Paradoxes of Everyday Life*

Unable to understand and reconcile the internal split she feels, a woman may experience justifiable anger— after all, she terminated a pregnancy to resolve one dilemma and is now left with a new one.

In order to free herself of this bind and resolve her anger, a woman must incorporate a fully fleshed out and whole "inner mother"—one who can both create and take life. Author and psychotherapist Maureen Murdock speaks of this mother archetype in the form of the ancient goddess Kali, a symbol of the feminine: "Kali Ma, the Hindu Triple Goddess of creation, preservation, and destruction, is known as the Dark Mother. She is the basic archetypal image . . . both giving life to her children and taking it away. She is the ancient symbol of the feminine portrayed in a thousand forms. . . . Kali's power has been forced underground just as many women's talents, skills, and energy have been suppressed as women acquiesce to gender roles that leave them depressed. . . ."

It is often difficult for a woman to recognize such a well-rounded inner force as Kali, yet when she has aborted she is faced with the reality of multiple powers. When the lesson of Kali is understood, a post-abortion woman knows that her decision to terminate a fetus, although perhaps a painful one, was not foreign to her instincts or the drive of the natural "inner mother." It may only be foreign to the culture in which she lives if that culture has resisted recognizing the multidimensional nature of the "inner mother."

The lesson of Kali also uncovers sources of a woman's anger. She may feel anger and rage for being unable to freely express the full range of her possibilities: to create life or to take life. She may feel anger when she is criticized for the power she naturally possesses. She may feel anger at being condemned when she exercises her power. She may feel anger at herself when she finds herself vacillating between knowing who she really is and pretending to be who society says she should be.

Murdock cautions women that recognizing their anger is only one step in healing that anger. She emphasizes that, "Kali's rage, when left unexpressed or unchannelled into creative forms, becomes the dark, devouring stagnation of life unlived."

In post–abortion terms, a woman's natural anger can turn into private pain or dark depression if it is not expressed. So, like the model of Kali, a woman must know her feelings, express them through word and/or action, and direct her energies into creating the life for which she ended her pregnancy. Marianne shares that she has done just that:

> I felt angry about my abortion and I wasn't going to let my life stagnate after going through it. I don't remember consciously thinking about it, but talking about this now, I recognize that I made an effort to make something positive come out of the pain.

Methods for expressing and channeling your anger will be discussed at the end of this chapter and in chapter 8, "The Process of Healing."

When a woman integrates more aspects of the "inner mother," she is able to understand that her decision to say "no" to a pregnancy is

Power can be taken, but not given. The process of the taking is empowerment in itself.

—Gloria Steinem

Outrageous Acts and Every-day Rebellions

as much a part of her nature as her decision to give life. If she feels anger, it must be honored and utilized and not misdirected in ways that are inappropriate for a healthy woman.

Exercise Four:

1. How have you considered the different "inner mother" parts of yourself? Nurturing? Boundary setting? Always loving? Withholding? Necessarily destructive?

2. What parts of your "inner mother" components are you the least comfortable with?

3. Who may have given you messages about having to be "all good" or "all loving"? Did you believe it? Do you still believe it?

4. How does your personal power to say "no" affect you? Is It hard? Easy? Scary?

5. Do you feel you have been criticized for being assertive?

6. How did having an abortion affect your life goals? Did you become motivated? More anxious? More confident? More reverent?

> If we go down into ourselves we find that we possess exactly what we desire.
>
> —Simone Weil
> *Gravity and Grace*

Once a woman has accepted that her feelings of anger are justified, exploring the sources related to her abortion experience can lead her to real peace.

Sources of Post-abortion Anger

No two women have post-abortion anger for exactly the same reasons. There are, however, commonly reported sources of anger. Women often feel anger toward themselves, their parents, the men who impregnated them and the doctors and clinic workers they encountered. Anger is also prominent among women who felt forced into an abortion, because it is a situation they never anticipated.

Anger at Themselves

The most readily identifiable anger women experience is the anger they feel toward themselves.

Trish's anger came after she exercised her power to say "no" to her pregnancy and later wished that she had not done so. Trish shares,

> When I look back, I regret my decision. My marriage was in good shape and our two kids were healthy. We are both lawyers, and I think we were just feeling overwhelmed with work and home life during that period. I would do it differently now. I was mad at myself for a long, long time.

> We could improve worldwide mental health if we acknowledged that parents can make you crazy.
>
> —Frank Zappa

Marianne, unlike Trish, was not mad over her choice to end her pregnancy, but was angry that she was not more responsible in planning to have her abortion earlier. By waiting until the last minute, she only increased her pain. Marianne said,

> I was so mad at myself! For only a few moments of sex, look at what I had to go through. I waited until the twelfth week, the last possible week. I was much more aware that there was a little life inside of me, as opposed to just tissue.

Susan was relentless in her anger and extremely ashamed of herself:

> I was feeling mean towards myself. "You're stupid. You're careless. You know you should have used birth control. You had sex with a married man." I was very critical of myself and reminded myself of how bad I was.

A woman's anger at herself is not always cut-and-dried, and it is often complicated by other relationships.

Anger at Parents

Many women who had experienced an unwanted pregnancy and abortion when they were young and still living at home felt anger toward their parents. The makeup of their specific emotions was as varied as their upbringing, but the one unifying factor was the conviction that their personal needs were not met in a time of crisis.

Stacy, like many women, feels she should have been better educated about birth control and sexual passion. Stacy was sixteen years old when she became pregnant:

> My mother and grandmother never took any responsibility for teaching me about birth control. I had to learn about sex in a hygiene class in high school. So I knew how to prevent pregnancy, but I didn't feel safe enough to go to my parents when I became sexually active and ask them to pay for birth control pills. They left it up to me, and I was a kid. At the clinic Mom just kept saying, "Don't do it! We're going to keep it and it is going to be mine." She was ready to take over my baby and still not talk to me about being a female or teach me about sexuality.

The most sympathetic of men never fully comprehend woman's concrete situation.
—Simone de Beauvoir
The Second Sex

Women were also angry if their parents had focused on achievements but neglected their daughters' emotional health. These women were frequently surprised by their own anger, because they knew how much their parents loved them and how hard their parents had worked in order to create a good home. Feeling anger was sometimes experienced as a betrayal, and was usually never shared. As Ellie relates about her high school pregnancy,

> The last thing I wanted to do was let my parents down. They pushed for me to be successful, as I was a first-generation American. I realize now that they pushed too much for my own good, but I didn't know it then. When I told my folks that I was pregnant, they became robot-like. They got me through it, but we never spoke about it.

Even when it was over, life was just supposed to go back to normal. I felt furious with them, and that was really hard. I was also angry because when I began dating again after my abortion, they still never spoke to me about sex. It took me years to realize that they just didn't know what to do or how to do it.

When home life was difficult, a young woman's pregnancy could become a personal nightmare although her anger might not surface until she was out of the house and free to feel her rage. Both of Suzanne's parents were alcoholics and "totally out of control." She kept her pregnancy a secret even at fifteen. When Suzanne was twenty-five her anger erupted:

> He who doesn't know anger doesn't know anything. He doesn't know the immediate.
>
> —Henri Michaux
> *Selected Writings*

My parents were miserable at being parents. I never told them I was pregnant because I knew what they were like. One drink and they became horribly abusive. It was too risky to share it because I knew it would come back at me. Angry? Damn right. They deserve it!

Often, when women tell their stories and are able to hear their own experience from beginning to end, they began to appreciate how normal their anger at their families was. They let go of the judgment that they were wrong to feel anger—it was natural for them to do so.

Anger at Men

As with the anger a woman may feel toward her parents, the anger she may feel toward the man who impregnated her is colored by their unique relationship. Sometimes women shared their anger and sometimes they chose silence in order to avoid emotional turmoil or the father's animosity:

I was so mad, really enraged at this man that I adored. We had talked about children, planned children, dreamt of children and then— poof!—he changed his mind. When I got pregnant I didn't even tell him.

—Anne

Oh, I felt angry all right! At myself for being so careless or stupid or misguided. And angry at my partner because he was completely inadequate and didn't rise to the occasion at all. I could have predicted that. It made me furious.

—Laura

> . . . a man never feels outraged unless in some respect he is at bottom right.
>
> —Victor Hugo
> *Les Misérables*

I was angry because my fiancé and I were just too old to be going through this in our thirties. We should have known better than to use "pulling out" as birth control.

—Meryl

I have irrational feelings of anger at my husband because he wanted a child. He told me the truth, that he wanted to be a father and he didn't pretend not to. Selfishly, I wanted him to support my choice. I wanted him to say, "I stand behind you, honey." I was angry that we wanted different things.

—Hallie

Jessica expresses a common reaction among post-abortion women. Her anger focuses on broader gender issues:

I feel angry that women carry this burden. I know men carry it too, but I think we have the pain—mostly. A lot of my women friends have had abortions, and the fathers never knew about it. So, those men never had a sleepless night looking at what so many of us have had to look at.

Abortion was illegal when I had mine. I was angry that I felt like an outlaw. A few years later I read an article about Jimmy Carter meeting with Catholic bishops to decide on the question of abortion. This really inflamed my rage. A bunch of men deciding what we were to do with our bodies. Especially a group of predominantly celibate men!

Anger at Doctors and Clinicians

Although the world
is full of suffering, it
is full also of the
overcoming of it.

—Helen Keller
Optimism

Doctors and clinicians sometimes become the focus of women's anger. Occasionally the women we spoke with encountered a judgmental physician who criticized them or addressed them in an abusive tone, and nurses who treated them with disinterest or even disdain:

I had enormous anger at the doctor, who was a creep. He walked into the room, never made eye contact or said hello to me. When I asked him a question, he was curt and abrupt.

—Cynthia

I hated being lined up with other women while the nurses chatted with each other about their Sunday night dates. There was a coldness and casualness that hurt. Shouldn't they have been paying attention to the patients?

—Ellie

I started to cry when the nurse began to insert the laminaria to dilate my cervix. She suddenly stopped and scolded me: "You need to sit up and pull yourself together. Go into the bathroom, get some tissues and throw some cold water on your face." I remember thinking, "You bitch."

—Sharon

Anger over an Unexpected Situation

Many times a woman feels anger over the unexpected nature of the abortion experience. It is an event she never anticipated and may have felt forced upon her. She never planned that her birth control would fail, that she would be date-raped, that her relationship would not withstand a pregnancy, or that she would ever be confronted with this enormous decision, which would eventually become a disturbing memory. When the rhythm of a woman's daily routine is destroyed and her personal history is unexpectedly rewritten, it is predictable that anger will ensue.

> Self-expression must pass into communication for its fulfillment.
> — Pearl Buck
> in *The Writer's Book,*
> Helen Hull

Lee was mad at the event:

There was no way my parents would have ever spoken to me again, had they known that I had gotten pregnant in high school. I wasn't adult enough to forge a life as a teenage mother on my own. And I didn't want the baby either. In order to remain a member of my family, I had to sacrifice something I hope to have sometime in the future—a child. I'm mad such a toll was required of me.

When Sharon received the news that she was carrying a fetus diagnosed with Down's syndrome, she faced an unplanned abortion. She shares,

This was the farthest thing from my mind even though my husband and I had discussed the fact that we would absolutely terminate a fetus that wasn't healthy. I was so sad and so angry that this pain had fallen upon our life. And the most unexpected anger was that I felt that I wasn't able to protect the child I was carrying.

The powerful love and affiliation Diane has with her husband, Henry, determined her choice to abort and simultaneously created disturbing anger as she felt forced into the situation.

With two kids and a husband who wasn't sure that he wanted another one or that our marriage would survive it, I didn't see a choice. Four days after the abortion we were at a friend's house and were singing along to his guitar. He sang a song about a little bear that dies, and I burst into tears. Although I never felt a hundred percent sure about having an abortion, I do believe it saved our marriage. I've felt angry and sad that our marriage required such a sacrifice.

> What we call failure is not the falling down, but the staying down.
>
> —Mary Pickford
>
> *Reader's Digest*

The choice Diane and Henry made served to sustain their marriage through a very difficult period in their lives. Although the momentous decision to terminate the fetus had to be made quickly, Diane took many months to work through her feelings of anger and loss about the whole situation.

Exercise Five:

1. Were you angry at yourself or other people at the time of your pregnancy and abortion?
2. How may your feelings of sadness or anger have been directed at yourself, at your parents or at the man involved?
3. Did you feel forced or pushed into a life event due to your pregnancy and abortion?
4. How might feeling forced have frustrated and angered you? Does it still?

Discerning Assertiveness from Aggressiveness

When women begin to express their anger, they are sometimes awkward in how they do it. A point to remember is that you have a right to take care of your needs, and a right to express your anger. It is also important to remember that other people have rights and personal boundaries too. Here are some basic guidelines:

Assertive Communication is when we express ourselves without threatening another person's rights and personal boundaries.

EXAMPLE OF ASSERTIVE COMMUNICATION: THIS IS A THREE STEP-PROCESS.

1. *When you* . . . [an action],
2. *I felt* . . . [an emotion],
3. *And what I would like is* . . . [your desire or need].

For example, Deneen might say to Danny:

"(I) Danny, *when you* left me when I got pregnant, (2) *I felt* angry, furious, hurt and abandoned. (3) *And what I would like is* an apology."

Or Mary might say to her mother:

"(I) Mom, *when you* helped me with my abortion but still didn't talk to me about sexual reproduction, (2) *I felt* confused, frustrated and angry. (3) *And what I would like is* for you to know that I will no longer depend on you for my emotional needs."

Notice that in this constructive three-step assertiveness model, the first statement only clarifies what the event is that you are referring to. The second step is an "I" statement about the emotions that you are feeling—not a thought. Some people make a mistake and say, "I feel that you are an idiot." This is not a statement of your feelings; this is *aggressive communication*. Make sure you state a feeling in order to ensure more constructive results. You can refer to the Feelings List in Appendix One if you need help identifying your emotions.

Aggressive communication is when we express our needs but transgress another person's rights and boundaries. This can cause the other person to become defensive or angry. It would be aggressive to say, in the second statement, "I feel you are an idiot." This is not a statement of your emotions; it is an attack on the other person. *Aggressive communication* can be vicious and hurtful, and everyone ends up feeling badly.

Stick with "I" statements regarding your feelings. No one can dispute your emotions. Your feelings are yours, and you have a right to them. If someone tries to tell you what you are feeling, or what you "should" be feeling, tell them, "There is no way you can know what I feel or what I 'should' feel, as you are not me. So, I am going to tell you again, 'I feel angry.' "

> Anger is our friend. Not a nice friend. Not a gentle friend. But a very, very loyal friend. . . . It will always tell us that it is time to act in our own best interests.
>
> —Julia Cameron
> *The Artist's Way*

Displaced and Misdirected Anger

Women tell us that they had anger they didn't directly manifest toward any past event. Instead, it displayed itself in displaced ways.

Sometimes, before a woman allows herself to identify and feel her anger, she finds herself "acting out" her feelings in disguised ways. Acting out serves as a cover-up for the real anger and can take many forms, including addictions.

> And I looked, and there was none to help; and I wondered that there was none to uphold: therefore mine own arm brought salvation unto me; and my fury, it upheld me.
>
> —Isaiah 63:5

Women have reported using eating disorders, alcohol and substance abuse, overspending, promiscuity, workaholism and perfectionism to deflect and mask their discomfort over many things—including abortion. For some women, it is more acceptable to take on a disorder than to be enraged. They may believe that no one likes an angry woman, so they choose a seemingly "harmless" acting out instead. At a party, such women can fade into the background, cultivating an eating disorder by munching chocolate chip cookies and then vomiting in the guest bathroom.

Another form of acting out is when a woman sets herself up for failure. If she imagines that she is "flawed," she can unconsciously construct ways to prove her negative self-concept is correct. She can oversleep and lose a job. She can ignore friends' needs and lose intimacy. Or she can give a great dinner party, serve a mediocre dish and then call the entire evening a failure. With these scenarios she can then say, "I never succeed because I'm undeserving." However genuine the emotions may seem, they are decoys for the real issue. It is up to the woman to determine if the real issue is anger or other resolved feelings about her abortion.

When a woman ignores her anger, other experiences can become magnified. Maggie was accepted by four out of the five graduate schools to which she applied. Yet, when she received her one rejection letter, she totally fell apart:

I was mad and felt sick at heart, as if I weren't good enough. It wasn't until much later, when I read back between the lines of my journal, that I realized I had been falling apart over an abortion I wasn't mourning.

Though Maggie kept ignoring her feelings of loss, they found new indirect ways to erupt in anger and self-judgments.

Emotional savvy prevents us from displacing our pain and tension. In the process of anger work, a woman must call it like it is: "I feel angry and depressed, and I think some of it has to do with my abortion."

Exercise Six:

1. How might you identify with any sort of "acting out"? Over-spending? An eating disorder? Promiscuity? Oversleeping? Smoking? Drinking? Drugs?

2. Did your acting out start or increase after your abortion? If so, how and when?

3. What things, other than your abortion, might be making you angry? Are you confusing various sources of your anger with your abortion? How?

> Once a human being has arrived on this earth, communication is the largest single factor determining what kinds of relationships he makes with others and what happens to him in the world about him.
>
> —Virginia Satir
> *Peoplemaking*

Ways to Constructively Express Anger

It is appropriate for you to feel and validate any anger you may have harbored as a result of your unwanted pregnancy and abortion—after all, your life was seriously interrupted. You have cause to be angry.

A challenging healing step occurs when you acknowledge and integrate dark parts of yourself that you may have previously deemed unacceptable. As poet Robert Bly says, a person must "eat [their] shadow" and gratefully recognize that she is not a combination of only "positive" qualities. Thus, rather than seeking emotional protection by playing a happy "Pollyanna," she confronts her darker Kali side and says to herself, "I feel angry about the whole mess. What I did does not fit my previous self-image, but that does not mean I would necessarily do it differently or that I am an unworthy human being." When anger is acknowledged and felt, it becomes necessary to express it in healthy ways.

Exercise Seven:

> I hate and love. You ask, perhaps, how can that be? I know not, but I feel the agony.
>
> —Catullus
> *Poems*

Along with writing your thoughts and feelings in the journal exercises, there are ways you can express your anger without hurting yourself or anyone else. Try the following:

1. Write a nasty letter and rip it up, flush it, bury it or burn it.
2. Write someone's name on the bottom of your shoes and stamp around.
3. Crush soda cans while saying things to a person in your imagination.
4. Beat pillows on a bed and holler about what is angering you.
5. Rip up old phone books and roar out your feelings.
6. Twist a towel and express what comes to mind.
7. Take a course in martial arts, go for a brisk walk or run, or play a vigorous game of your favorite sport.

Try the above, or make up new ideas to physically express your anger in healthy ways.

Over time, a woman may come to realize that the split she feels between her desired "all-good" self and any other self-traits, such as the "destructive" aspect, has the potential to incite self-directed anger if not accepted as part of being human. She may be able to transcend Emily Dickinson, who felt

> . . . a Cleaving in my Mind—
> As if my Brain had split—
> I tried to match it—Seam by Seam—
> But could not make them fit.

When a woman recognizes the sources of her anger and realizes that the feeling itself is a normal, valid emotion to which she is entitled, her awareness broadens and she becomes more whole. Paradoxically, she also becomes less angry.

The healthy expression of anger is all part of closure on post-abortion pain for the sake of your emotional and physical well-being.

Parts of Ourselves Are in the Shadows

There are many parts of our own character that we do not know. This is normal. It is as if those parts are in the shadows. When we shine the light of insight on those shadow parts, the light may illuminate some knowledge, but we also see that new shadows appear. The shining of the light keeps giving us more and more insight about ourselves, but the process is never complete. This is a natural part of being whole. Even though we may have resistance strategies against personal change, due to habit, convention or social pressure, it is our job to question what is scary about abortion acceptance and overcome the resistance—to keep shining the light on our very exclusive self.

No one else has the same unique inner life as any other person. Martha Graham said, "There is a vitality, a life force, an energy, a quickening, that is translated through you into action, and because there is only one of you in all time, this expression is unique. And if you block it, it will never exist through any other medium and will be lost."

Healing comes in the conscious search. Arrival is in the journey.

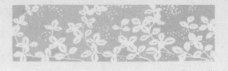

Chapter Six
Spirituality and Religion

"All inquiries carry with them some element of risk."
—Carl Sagan
Broca's Brain

When a woman travels from conception to abortion, she realizes she can both create and take potential life. This awakening may be distressing if she views herself as a religious or spiritual woman who regards all life as sacred—even potential life.

When we speak of "spirituality" in this chapter, we refer to a deep passion for life, a feeling of wonderment, awe and intangible fascination for the powers that make the sun rise and a flower bloom, and a connectedness between one's personal self and the universe. Spirituality might be thought of as that force that wants all things to be the most they can be: a caterpillar the most beautiful butterfly it can be, a bud the most marvelous flower it can be and a transcendent awareness that can make you the most that you can be.

When we speak of "religion" we refer to organizations with laws and rituals within which a person hopes to experience their spirituality—Christianity, Judaism, Catholicism, Buddhism, etc.

Spirituality might be thought of as the "contents" that a person pours into the "container" of an organized religion.

In a time of crisis, an individual either flees or takes an action toward resolving the problem. If the spiritual or religious woman is faced with an unwanted pregnancy, something from which she cannot flee, she may instinctively react and choose to resolve her crisis by having an abortion.

Sometimes the pressure of limited time in which to abort allows the woman to only briefly examine her beliefs. Only after the fetus has been terminated may the full impact of her decision begin to plague her. But it is too late to reconsider the decision to abort. Eventually she may come to feel stuck, wedged between her previous spiritual precepts and her personal needs.

> Spirit is an invisible force made visible in all life.
>
> —Maya Angelou
> *Wouldn't Take Nothing For My Journey Now*

Spirituality and religion may converge at times, and at times they may be diametrically opposed. If you are a woman with spiritual pain, you might consider the possible interplay between spirituality, religion and a past abortion. The peace of many post-abortion women is a spiritual journey, for others it is a religious one and for still others, it is a spiritual *and* a religious journey.

The Spiritual Woman

Spirituality for the post-abortion woman may include many elements. Certainly the relationship to her body and her ability to create life is a significant aspect.

Early Feelings of the Spiritual

Although civilized society mostly overlooks the significance of a girl's awakening fertility, there is a stirring within the girl's personal psyche very early on. Whether she is consciously aware of it or not, the fact remains that any pubescent girl is able to create a human life. But with no designated rituals to educate or celebrate the shift in a female's identity from child to life-giver, the uninitiated young woman is at a disadvantage and is often unprepared to name the source of the spiritual waves that begin with the earliest signs of puberty.

Maturing Spirituality

As a woman matures and develops a sense of the spiritual, she may find herself understanding things simply by opening herself to a guiding power within her psyche. Some women believe that these spiritual feelings arise from a connection to the collective unconscious, a place greater than the individual self that has been passed down over centuries, carbon-copied into DNA matter and slipped into the cells of human beings. Spiritual women have reported that a sense of "something greater" is always with them, and that they are usually able to tap into it.

> There will always be arguments based on spiritual or ethical beliefs to convince an individual of the rightness or wrongness of abortion . . .
>
> —Charles A. Gardner
> "Is an Embryo a Person?"
> *The Nation*

Spirituality and Abortion

A woman is sometimes pained by her spiritual beliefs when faced with healing a crisis like a past abortion. She may feel awe at the realization that she can give life. And, in like manner, she may be stunned by the enormity of the paradoxical truth that she is able to take life. If a woman did not want a child, or felt that the time was not right, she may have acted against what she had previously defined as spiritual. Her work is to find self-acceptance within her present spiritual beliefs, or to redefine her beliefs to include the reality of her action.

Rather than conception being associated with life-giving, conception, when coupled with abortion, becomes associated with conflict. For a woman to simultaneously view herself as a "creator" and a "destroyer" can give way to confusion and vital questioning of her character, her moral convictions and her identity as a spiritual woman.

The split asks that a woman reexamine components of her spirituality, understand that spirituality encompasses her appreciation of all life—including her own—and that maturity is finding her own truth within a situation. The reconciliation asks that she not see life as an all-or-nothing proposition like the youngster who still makes judgments as black and white. It asks that she gain the ability to handle concepts such as "good rules don't always apply." This is the maturity of inner work that any crisis can invite. If we can grow from pain, it is not wasted.

As a post-abortion woman, Melanie relates her understanding of the spiritual:

> The spiritual paradox about my abortion is that I respect life, be it a person or a plant. I respected my own life and all life so much, I chose to rid myself of the tissue that could have been a baby so that my life could go forward. At that time, it wouldn't have been a good life for a child.

Melanie's spiritual relationship to nature speaks of her trust in what author Clarissa Pinkola Estes calls the Life/Death/Life cycle. Melanie says,

> I always notice that nature renews herself, spring always follows winter. A spring came after my abortion. My life moved forward.

Anne relates her experience thus:

> I have always described myself as spiritual, and my abortion was a catalyst to test the strength of that conviction. I felt that to have an unwanted child would be the ultimate example of a disregard for the sanctity of life. To not protect something so sacred would contradict my philosophy of life. This is not to say that my choice was easy or made without guilt—but my spiritual belief system gave me comfort at a time when I felt great sadness.

Melanie and Anne delicately operated from a spiritual basis to reach their decisions to abort—for their or their families' betterment.

> Spirituality leaps where science cannot yet follow, because science must always test and measure, and much of reality and human experience is immeasurable.
>
> —Starhawk
> *The Spiral Dance*

They were not callous or uncaring. In making, and later in reviewing, their decisions to abort, they considered their natural tendencies to care for others first. They realized that recognition of their own needs was neither unfeminine nor unacceptable. They acted to further their life course in spite of an unwanted pregnancy. They recognized that they had the latent ability to take life (or potential life) and painfully exercised that option. They felt that choosing for their life's desires was spiritual in itself.

> Where is there dignity unless there is honesty?
>
> —Marcus Tullius Cicero

Exercise One:

1. Define your sense of spirituality.

2. Do you relate to spirituality on an everyday basis? How?

Women's Relationship to Life and Loss

For centuries women have spoken to one another about life. They have confided the tiniest details about the births of their children. They have shared the news of children born to siblings and to their own children.

Women have also spoken to one another about death: in quiet moments over a back fence, sitting in front of a fire, walking on a trail in the mountains, or on the phone. They have sought comfort from one another when grandparents, parents, spouses and children have passed away. They have held one another in mourning after miscarriages. And they have cried together over abortions.

We have already seen that women as "creators of life" is a far easier concept for society to acknowledge than women as "creators of loss." There has been an abundance of media images to support this stereotype. Movies are filled with male heroes with a gun or hatchet who face a foe and must make the decision to take a life or let the poor person go. The audience can accept the male in his guise as the "rock 'em, sock 'em," "shoot 'em up" guy who has the right or duty to kill. It is proof of his virility. But there is little cultural support for a woman when she chooses to terminate a pregnancy. Not in the movies, and not in real life. And so, when a woman decides to abort, it is a very private experience that she alone must learn to value as right for her.

3. What questions challenged your sense of spirituality at the time of your abortion?

4. What spiritual questions about your abortion continue to linger until today?

5. Make a list of what you are confident about in your personal spirituality.

6. Using the above list, decide which specific assumptions, if any, you may have to reexamine in order to find peace.

7. Were you previously affiliated with a specific religion? How might remnants of that doctrine still affect your spiritual beliefs?

Continue to read the following sections and consider the information that is pertinent to you.

The Religious Woman

> We think of Divine Oneness as feeling the intent and the emotion of beings—not as interested in what we do as why we do it.
>
> —Marlo Morgan
> *Mutant Message Down Under*

Women across the religious spectrum frequently tell of experiencing pre- and post-abortion emotional pain. They may be Orthodox or Reform, Christian or Jewish, Moslem, Buddhist, Hindu or agnostic. They may worship outside a religious sanctuary or attend a church or a synagogue. However, neither the religious belief system women embrace, nor the manner in which they express that philosophy, can determine the degree of spiritual conflict they will feel over their abortion. And these factors cannot predict the ease with which their spiritual conflict will be resolved.

Devoutly religious women from denominations that ban abortion often fear they may struggle with misgivings about their past abortions for many years. Although resolving their pain can be especially difficult if their religion is inflexible regarding abortion, their dilemma is clear: they did something that is unacceptable in the eyes of God.

Even women who feel a less rigid religious identification are sometimes amazed by their discomfort. Although their lives have never been guided by strong religious doctrines, they may now find themselves worrying, "Will God punish me for ending my pregnancy?" "Will my future children by punished for my abortion?"

If you are a woman who feels uncertain about the connections between abortion and religion, or if you are sure that God looks upon abortion as a sin, it will be helpful to sort out your personal sense of the spiritual from the rules that your religion offers.

To help you identify the presence of any conflicts you may feel, look at the following list and take note of your response to each phrase:

> And what is religion, you might ask. It's a technology of living.
>
> —Toni Cade Bambara
> *The Salt Eaters*

- I have no religious pain over my abortion.
- I believe that abortion is killing.
- I trust that God understands why I aborted.
- I know that God will never forgive me for having an abortion.
- My choice to abort has had no impact on my belief in God or God's love for me.
- I am not sure if I believe in God, but I fear that my abortion would not be condoned by God.
- I would like to receive forgiveness from a priest, minister or rabbi for having an abortion.
- I don't know if I have religious pain over my abortion.

Acknowledging that you are carrying religious pain over your abortion, if that is true for you, is an important step in resolving your unrest. Understanding the nature of your conflict comes next.

Religion and Abortion

Family therapist Robin Schwartz Kapper, whose practice includes pre-abortion counseling, tells us that sometimes a woman feels religious conflict while making plans to abort. Rather than focusing on the enormous issue of religion, Schwartz Kapper says, "Women want to examine their pregnancies by looking at more manageable and practical concerns, such as, 'Can I adequately support and care for this child?' " Although a religious conflict may still remain and need to be addressed, most often women possess the conscious knowledge that they had sound practical reasons for terminating their pregnancies.

When a post-abortion religious woman begins to explore her conflict she may find that it is not easily resolved. If she respects her decision to abort, is she saying that God is wrong? How can she honor God without believing that she has committed a terrible sin? By having an abortion, has she abandoned her baby and abandoned God as well? Has she stayed with God and with herself but abandoned her religion?

> Religion controls inner space; inner space controls outer space.
>
> —Zsuzsanna E. Budapest
> "Self Blessing Ritual"
> in *Womanspirit Rising,*
> Carol P. Christ
> and Judith Plaskow

If a woman fears that she has contradicted the will of God by aborting a fetus from her womb, a deep hurt may open within her psyche. How she reacts to that wound is unpredictable, but this pain has the potential to send shock waves reverberating through her inner life: her self-esteem may be affected; she may worry that her immortal soul is tarnished; she may fear for her future well-being; she may be riddled with guilt and shame; she may doubt her ability to maintain her faith; she may confess her "sin" and become devoutly religious; she may worry for the safety of her future offspring, whom, she fears, God will harm.

Trapped in conflict, the religious woman needs to make a decision. She can either live with long-term fear, guilt and depression, asking herself over and over again, "Have I made a terrible mistake?" "Will I be punished for this decision?" or she can explore the roots of her conflict, define her personal spirituality and move toward mature resolution.

The Roots of Religious Conflict

The roots of religious conflict rest not only in a woman's personal religious background, but also in the messages she has gleaned from abortion's history as a religious issue and a source of ongoing political and theological debate.

Religious teachings impart moral values that offer guidelines for behavior. They may take the form of a rabbi's interpretation of a biblical passage, the doctrine proclaimed by the Catholic papacy, lessons taught in a Sunday school class, or even a parent's reading of a Bible story to a child at bedtime.

> God enters by a private door into every individual.
> —Ralph Waldo Emerson
> "Intellect"
> *Essays, First Series*

A woman who terminates a pregnancy is usually aware of the ways in which her religion regards abortion; she is also aware of how her family, friends and the members of her religious community would view her decision in light of their own spiritual convictions. When a woman trusts that she is supported in her choice, she may feel little or no spiritual unrest. But when she senses that there would be opposition to her choice, or if she has already experienced opposition directly, she is often left with religious conflict and emotional pain.

Connie was raised in a moderately observant Catholic family in the Midwest. Although she regularly attended church as a child, she stopped going as an adult. She believed a single woman who was sexually active and using birth control could not, in good conscience, be worshiping as a Catholic.

When Connie became pregnant at twenty-nine, with a man she had just begun dating, she experienced feelings of religious guilt. At the news of her pregnancy, she confided in her mother who, over the years, had become increasingly involved in the Church. Connie tells us,

> My mother was just amazing when I told her that I was going to have an abortion. I explained my reasons, and she never once disagreed with me. She told me she would have made a different choice for herself, but was supportive of the decision I was making for myself. She was a source of love and support throughout the entire ordeal and even reassured me that God would never hate me.

Her mother's ability to separate her religious doctrine from her daughter's needs was a great gift for Connie. Nevertheless, the months following her abortion were sometimes difficult for Connie. She began to have problems with alcohol as well as bulimia, an eating disorder that she had thought was long under control. She entered psychotherapy and talked about everything but her unplanned pregnancy, which, in her mind, had been resolved with its termination.

Nearly a year after the day of her abortion, Connie was visiting her parents and accompanied her mother to a mall:

> I was standing in line at a department store, and just behind me was a woman about my age holding a baby. I was watching the baby and the baby was looking back at me, and it hit me—a wave of overwhelming guilt and grief. It was about God and sin and being a Catholic woman who had sex outside of marriage and got pregnant and had an abortion. It was about having done it all wrong; at least it was that way in my mind at the time.

Listen, God love everything you love—and a mess of stuff you don't.
—Alice Walker
The Color Purple

Connie, having found a Catholic counselor whom she trusted to be impartial and with whom she felt emotionally safe, was able to explore her personal religious conflict. Connie's counselor told her, "Our Church has an obligation to state what is believed to be right and wrong. However, not everyone can choose what the Church deems to be right. The Church must set up an ideal, but each individual must reconcile that ideal with their individual preferences." Connie realized that neither the comfort she received from her mother nor her use of substances and addictive behaviors could eradicate the spiritual unrest she felt. At the time of our interview, Connie told us that she had gained a great deal of insight into her conflict. She explained that working through her feelings required that she reexamine her sexuality and sort through what she believed was true about her body, from what she was told was incontestable. She also said that she still thought of herself as Catholic and began to attend church once again, even though her personal spirituality differed from the Church's to some degree. She believed that she could be deeply religious and validate her own spirituality and sexuality at the same time. Connie tells us,

> At the present, I feel a certain amount of "spiritual comfort" in that I have some self-forgiveness and self-acceptance. I have reached an inner resolution about my abortion.

She emphasizes that her resolution "isn't tied up with a neat little bow," but that it is her truth. It also allows her to reinstate her faith.

I cannot prove this but I suspect that abortion must have been practiced from time immemorial.

—Irene Claremont de Castillejo
Knowing Woman

Exercise Two:

Whether you are a woman who has remained influenced by the religious ideology you were taught as a child or a woman who has embraced a spiritual belief system in adulthood, your recovery may ask that you explore your conflict by considering the following questions:

1. What were the religious messages you were taught as a child regarding abortion?
2. What were your religious beliefs concerning abortion when you terminated your pregnancy?
3. What are your religious beliefs concerning abortion today?
4. How has your choice to end a pregnancy influenced your view of yourself as a religious woman?
5. Do you believe that your religious philosophy and your choice to abort are compatible?
6. If your religion takes no stand on abortion but you feel conflict, what beliefs do you hold about God and abortion? Where did these beliefs come from?

7. If you have recognized the presence of religious messages that conflict with your choice, how have they made you feel?

Through the possible identification of religious messages that contradict your choice, no matter how great or small they may be, you are defining aspects of your conflict. If you feel discord but cannot trace it to your personal religious background, you might be responding to other individual misgivings or even to powerful media messages about abortion as a controversial issue in society today.

> All major religions are patriarchal. They were founded to spread or buttress male supremacy—which is why their gods are male.
>
> —Marilyn French
> *The War Against Women*

Abortion as an Historic Religious Controversy

Women, whether directly affected by the religious controversy on abortion or not, often find themselves victims of its fury when faced with an unplanned pregnancy. Women with strongly held religious philosophies may feel enhanced pain when they terminate a pregnancy, and women for whom abortion has never been a religious issue may internalize the outer world's conflict and feel it as their own.

Where abortion was once seen as an issue apart from a woman's relationship with God, today the two have frequently become inseparable for many people. To appreciate the intensity of the outer world's impact on the emotional well-being of post-abortion women, it is helpful to understand the development of abortion as a religious issue.

The History of Abortion

In ancient times, before the Judeo-Christian era, Mother Earth was the symbolic giver of life. Many peoples honored her fertility by worshiping the goddess. When she was pleased, her crops were bountiful; when she was ill tempered, her crops were sparse.

Just as the goddess was deemed to determine when the harvest would grow, author Judith Arcana believes that it was also a woman's prerogative to decide if her fertile womb would create life or if she would abort.

That a woman was able to create and release a fetus was not regarded as blasphemous. Termination was seen as a woman's choice and honored as a sorrowful one.

Over time, worship of the goddess diminished as advances in herding and commerce took hold and communities became less reliant upon Mother Earth to provide sustenance. The goddess was redefined as "pagan," although many theologians believe she found her way into Western religions as Mary in Christianity and as the Shekinah in Judaism.

> Abortion was known and discussed even in Talmudic times; there were even specified rituals for a woman who had undergone one.
>
> —Susan Weidman Schneider
> *Jewish and Female*

With the demise of the goddess came the rise of the patriarchy and a changing world for women and their reproductive rights.

Abortion and the Rise of the Patriarchy

The patriarchy secured its foothold four to five thousand years ago. As male gods with patriarchal values emerged, according to historian Marija Gimbutas, the importance of the goddess was inevitably diminished and a woman's revered status in the community was reduced.

The fate of a woman's reproductive life, as with most aspects of her existence, became male domain. The patriarchy substantiated its power by viewing conception as a spiritual function favoring man over woman. Some cultures saw a man's semen as an extension of his soul. The early Greeks believed that semen contained multiple fully formed tiny human beings, while a woman's uterus merely incubated the homunculi to viability. Author Barbara Walker points out, "If the fetus he conceived were destroyed, then surely the man himself would suffer spiritual injury" unless he himself chose for destruction of the fetus.

The early Catholic Church regarded abortion as wrong for the sins it hid, adultery and fornication, but not wrong in itself. In A.D. 1150, a canon law decreed that abortion was murder only if the fetus was formed—at forty days if it was male and ninety days if it was female. Very little changed in the Church's stand toward abortion for eight hundred years.

In 1917, Catholic women began to lobby for their reproductive freedom. In response, the Church, under the order of Pope Pius IX, directed that abortion be punished by excommunication. In 1968, activist women forced the issue once again, resulting in Pope Paul VI forbidding contraception and all abortion. In 1974, one year after abortion had been legalized in the United States, the Vatican declared that abortion, carried out at any time in a pregnancy and for any reason, constituted murder; this continues to be the Vatican's stance.

> We live in a true chaos of contradicting authorities, an age of conformism without community, of proximity without communication.
>
> —Germaine Greer
> *The Female Eunuch*

Fundamentalist Christian groups, framing abortion as a universal moral issue, became a vocal influence in North America beginning in the 1970s. By defining themselves as religious *and* political, and supporting like-minded candidates, many attempted to enforce their philosophical views through governmental legislation. Simply stated, they considered abortion to be both a religious and a criminal offense: the taking of life. Their goals included making abortion illegal once again.

Jewish women have faced a far less oppressive religious force than have many Christian and Catholic women. Abortion was sanctioned in the early days of the Jewish religion and, aside from the strict Orthodoxy, which disallows abortion unless an abnormal fetus endangers the mother's life, has remained accepted throughout Judaic history and among its peoples. The position held by contemporary Reform and Conservative Jews in the United States was stated by the American Jewish Congress in 1972: "Those who find abortion unacceptable as a matter of religious conviction or conscience are free to hold and live by their beliefs, but should not seek to impose such beliefs, by government actions, on others."

Judaism's stance supports statistics showing that only 15 percent of Jewish women object to abortion, while 50 percent of Protestant women and 67 percent of Catholic women are strongly opposed to the termination of a pregnancy. Researchers Zolese and Blacker conducted a study which suggested that post-abortion "Roman Catholics experience more guilt than Protestants, Protestants more guilt than Jews."

In contrast to those religious groups that strongly oppose abortion and sometimes regard it as an appropriate political cause, numerous Christian churches and other organizations have less stringent beliefs. The Religious Coalition for Reproductive Choice, composed of Christian, Jewish, Catholic, and other groups, sees abortion as a woman's personal prerogative not as a political or religious issue.

> Jupiter is slow looking into his notebook, but he always looks.
>
> —Zenobius
> *Sententiae*

The Impact of the Religious Controversy on a Woman

Today's women have been impacted by society's controversial thoughts and feelings on abortion as a religious or political issue. They have heard heated arguments on the subject, seen marches on the country's capital and listened to candidates debate.

Some women, witnessing society's upheaval, have held to their personal religious truths. Other women have felt an intensified confusion, and still others have experienced a degree of unrest they had never anticipated as they attempt to process and assimilate the external world of conflict.

Janet defined herself as a liberal Jewish woman who felt a clear separation between her choice to terminate her pregnancy and her religious and political leanings. Nevertheless, her abortion sensitized her to the controversy in the external world. She told us,

> I don't particularly care what anyone thinks about my decision to abort, and their opinions have not made me question my belief in God or my politics. I have always been very aware of the religious

debate on abortion, but since my own abortion, I have become even more aware of other people's beliefs and that they are far more emotional about the whole issue than I am.

Exercise Three:

Consider the following questions and the ways in which your feelings about your abortion have been impacted by the religious controversy in society.

> Concern should drive us into action and not into a depression.
>
> —Karen Horney
> *Self-Analysis*

1. How might society's conflict have influenced your feelings about your own abortion?
2. How do you feel about the religious and political conflict surrounding abortion? Have your feelings changed over time?
3. Do you consider abortion to be either a religious or a political issue?
4. What are your thoughts and feelings about the religious and political debate on abortion? Have you expressed that opinion either publicly or privately?

The Fear of Retribution

Living with the fear that one has defied God by choosing to abort a fetus has far-reaching psychological implications for many women. Well-designed psychological studies concur. In their research, Congleton and Calhoun concluded that the post-abortion women who "had significantly higher scores on initial stress responses and religiosity were more often currently affiliated with conservative churches."

Devoutly religious post-abortion women may suffer with the recurring thought that they will be punished by God, and agnostic women may also feel haunted by vague concerns they cannot identify.

Charlotte had no strong religious affiliation, but she still worried that God, if there was a God, would retaliate against her personally:

I live with the dread that somehow I will have to pay for this decision. I'm not sure how that will happen. But sometimes when something bad happens, I worry that this is the payback. And when something good happens, I worry that it will be taken away. Maybe my constant paranoia is the punishment. Then again, maybe there is no punishment at all.

> By being obedient to external requirements over a long period of time, [a person] loses his real powers of ethical, responsible choice.
>
> —Rollo May
> *Man's Search for Himself*

Other women worry that God will punish them by preventing them from ever bearing children, or by inflicting their future children with birth defects. Wendy, who was reared in a Reform Jewish home with virtually no religious traditions, says,

I felt like I would be punished for the rest of my life. I felt that I wouldn't be able to have children or, if I did, something might be wrong with them. I felt they'd have problems because of what I've done, that this thing would bother me for rest of my life!

Vicky's devout upbringing left her fearful of the potential for religious backlash as well. She has not been a practicing Catholic since her teens, but at the time of her abortion she could not shake the tenets of her childhood. Vicky worried that the fetus she aborted might be damned. She says,

I remember saying a prayer after my abortion because I didn't know if babies had souls. From what I remembered of Catholicism, if a baby dies without being baptized, it goes to purgatory. I just hoped it would be given another chance and not be out in purgatory because of what I had done.

Vicky shares that in the twenty years since her abortion, she has sometimes prayed that God would "send this baby's soul to somebody else who will love and care for it." Vicky's prayers give her solace and helped her to grieve her loss.

Exercise Four:

If you have experienced the fear of retribution, stop and consider how that fear has touched your life.

1. Do you believe God might punish you personally? In what ways?
2. Do you worry that He will punish you through harming your offspring? How might He do that?

Seeking Forgiveness from External Authority Figures

> I want the freedom to carve and chisel my own face, to staunch the bleeding with ashes, to fashion my own gods out of my entrails.
>
> —Gloria Anzaldua
> *Borderlands/La Frontera:*
> *The New Mestiza*

Because many religious women are reluctant to forgive themselves for choosing an abortion over adoption or keeping the baby, they can remain trapped in confusion. In their endeavor to sort things out and find acceptance, they may be uncertain whether to empower their own inner authority, contact an external authority figure or both.

For many women, seeking forgiveness from external authority figures is not done simply because they can't forgive themselves. They may want to express themselves through the rituals offered within their religious framework. Two such rituals are the "sacrament of reconciliation" in the Catholic Church and the "mizuko kuyo" or "water child" ritual in Buddhism. For some women, there is great value in rituals that offer outward expression of heartfelt pain, conflict or guilt. In chapter 8 there are suggestions and examples of personal rituals which might be helpful whether a woman is religious, spiritual, neither or both.

When a woman seeks outer authority figures to calm the tension inside her, she may find constructive, non-guilt-inducing help. She also, however, runs the risk of reinforcing the old belief that her personal judgments are inadequate. Ellen, raised in the Lutheran church, found her pastor's help to be a steppingstone to her acceptance of her abortion. She says,

> I called a church to talk to a pastor after my abortion because I really wanted to get answers from somebody who knows God the best.

Ellen found that her pastor's words were a helpful beginning. Over time she found that she needed to do additional inner work to integrate her abortion experience.

Having others tell a woman that "God will forgive you" may help to relieve her stress, but unless she has truly resolved her feelings internally, it is only a matter of time before her doubts and conflicts return. As Vicky relates,

> I spent forty-five minutes talking to a priest about my abortion. He told me that he thought I was far harder on myself than God would ever be and that God was very forgiving. At the time I felt relief that he had said this, but it took me another year before I believed it myself.

Turning to others for total absolution may initially feel appropriate, but it is just one step, in several, that a woman takes toward personal resolution. As author and psychologist Rollo May explains, unquestioning obedience to an external authority figure causes one to lose the ability to make individual moral and responsible choices.

It takes courage for a religious woman to consider forgiving herself when she fears that she might have angered God. Doing so can feel like another sacrilegious act—"just like my abortion." It may go

---

We are not born all at once, but by bits. The body first, and the spirit later; and the birth and growth of the spirit, in those who are attentive to their own inner life, are slow and exceedingly painful.

—Mary Antin
The Promised Land

against her firm belief that only an external authority figure—such as a priest, a rabbi, a minister or a pastor—can offer her valid forgiveness. It is important for this woman to recognize that the authority figure's forgiveness may only partially serve her if she still experiences spiritual unrest. It is then an opportunity for her to look to her own truth and forgive herself. It is her chance to recognize and develop a unique spirituality that offers deep personal peace. In this way, she defines her own spirituality within the "container" of her religion.

> If we would have new knowledge, we must get a whole world of new questions.
> —Susanne K. Langer
> *Philosophy in a New Key*

There is no precise religious "high ground" after an abortion for the religious woman. Her self-imposed moral dilemma can be crushing and cause immense guilt, or it can lead to self-respect and a greater understanding of her inner truth. For the religious woman, the path to resolution must include "forgiveness." Her personal forgiveness may not always fit comfortably within her religious doctrine, but it can induce maturation of her own spirituality.

Taking control of one's life and supporting one's decisions is an act of strength that can reinforce a woman's inner authority. As Sharon, who aborted a Down's syndrome fetus, says,

> I never went to talk to a rabbi about what the Jewish faith thinks about abortion because, honestly, I don't care. I believe that this decision was based upon what I personally regard as moral, humane and spiritual. So, I am not bothered by what other people might think. It was a private decision, and God and I know why I made it.

If you have unhealed spiritual wounds, you might consider turning to an unbiased authority figure for counseling. You might also turn to yourself, as you are the authority figure who knows what is right for you in your life.

Healing the Wound

It can be challenging for a religious woman, uncomfortable with a past abortion, to remain within her church or synagogue. She may struggle with her efforts to redefine her image of God—from punishing to forgiving, from angry to loving, from uncompromising to accepting—in order to take the power of healing and self-forgiveness into her own hands.

i found god in my-
self
& i loved her
i loved her fiercely.
—Ntozake Shange
For Colored Girls Who Have
Considered Suicide/
When the Rainbow Is Enuf

There is predictable hesitancy when one is asked to examine and explain one's religious identity, because the very nature of religion often demands obedience and acceptance based upon blind faith. To challenge any aspect of that faith is to question the comfort it is intended to bring. A religious woman may not risk such questioning unless a strong individual act, such as an abortion, has led her to experience significant spiritual unrest.

In order to begin the formidable task of resolving her confusion, it is helpful for a woman to step back from what she has been taught in her religious life and from society at large. She must turn down the volume on her emotions and initially guide herself with her intellect. From this less tumultuous place, she can begin the hard work of examining herself and her religion. From this dispassionate place she can begin to discover a spiritual path that will enhance her individual dignity and self-worth, and very possibly combine her previous teachings with new insights.

If you consider yourself a religious woman, you started your healing work the moment you began reading this book. You may have already recognized uncomfortable religious feelings arising from your choice to abort and acknowledged that you are a spiritual woman with pain. You then may have felt some need to explore your distress. Exercises 2, 3 and 4 in this chapter offered you the possibility to examine the

sources of the religious conflict in your life, how society's religious controversy has impacted your well-being and your fears of retribution. If you
skipped these exercises, consider doing them now. You also have had the
opportunity to weigh personal responsibility for reconciling your religious conflict rather than turning to outside authority figures. Reading
these pages and working the exercises is a testament to that pursuit.

Now you are asked to respectfully deconstruct and reconstruct
the specific religious doctrines that conflict with your past
abortion. This may feel like a threatening challenge, but it
is an immediately helpful option if you are to genuinely
free yourself of untenable conflict. To arrive at a place of
psychological balance does not necessitate abandoning
your religion or abandoning God; it suggests integrating
the general precepts of your religious life with your even
more thoroughly explored, individually experienced spirituality. In
this way, you may be able to meld your spiritual and religious philosophies.

> As truly as God is our Father, so truly is God our Mother.
>
> —Julian of Norwich
> *Revelations of Divine Love*

A religious system is most constructive when it provides support
to your search for self-worth, affirms your genuine values and offers
you a sense of community.

Exercise Five:

The work of respectfully reexamining and deconstructing your religious beliefs is
possible. It requires that you understand what you have been taught in your
spiritual life.

Reconstructing a religious belief system asks that you open your mind to
new ideas and consider disregarding old ones that may be presented as univer-
sally correct for everyone, but that don't respect you.

The following questions are meant to point you in a "constructive" direction. Do not expect to arrive at new conclusions immediately; this entire process
takes careful thought and time.

1. What are your spiritual needs as a post-abortion woman?

2. How has your religious belief system strengthened your sense of dignity and self-worth?

3. Do you feel that your religious belief system has allowed you to form your own value system, even if some of your views do not agree with the teachings of the religion?

4. In what ways have you been supported in your personal beliefs?

> God ain't a he or a she, but a It.
>
> —Alice Walker
> *The Color Purple*

5. In what ways has your particular religious organization made it easy or difficult for you to form your own values and moral code?

6. Can you receive healing and acceptance for your abortion in your religious system without undue acquiescence or guilt?

7. Since your abortion, have you felt pressure to admit wrongdoing even if you don't believe your decision was wrong?

8. If you decide to remain within your religious belief system, are you willing to find a place to worship where you will feel supported and respected for your personal choices?

9. If you decide to reject your religious belief system, what will you replace it with?

10. If you truly regret having aborted, where might you find a place in your religious belief system that compassionately forgives you without undue condemnation?

Exercise Six:

Write a letter to God or whatever force you have chosen as your concept of a higher power. In that letter you might want to include the following:

1. Explain the reasons for your decision to terminate your pregnancy.

2. Write about why that decision may have been in your best interests. Also write about why the abortion may have been in the best interests of the fetus as well.

3. Write about why that decision may not have been in your best interests. What have you learned about your best interests since then?

4. Explain why you felt this was the best decision you could make at the time.

5. Tell God what you need from Him or Her.

Exercise Seven:

Write a letter of forgiveness to yourself from your own Inner Authority. Do so with love and compassion. Once again, take time and recall why you thought and felt that your choice was correct at the time—for yourself and for the fetus you aborted. Begin your letter:

> "Dear _____[your name]."

And, after you finish, sign it:

> "With forgiveness, Your Inner Authority."

> New gods arise when they are needed.
>
> —Josephine Johnson
> *Sisters of the Earth*
> Lorraine Anderson, ed.

Exercise Eight (Optional):

Having a spiritual sanctuary within which to worship, and religious leaders to turn to for guidance, is a wonderful resource. While going to outer authority figures to replace your own inner authority can lessen your personal strength, using them for additional support can offer comfort and solace. Feel free to interview spiritual people—priests, pastors, ministers or rabbis—who offer more than the representation of a vengeful God. They do exist within your chosen religion. A search will allow you to find them.

As a religious woman works to create a balance between her religion's doctrines and her spiritual convictions, she can begin to accept her abortion.

Connie tells us about her struggle to come to terms with her choice:

I have spent a great deal of time recently just listing the reasons why I chose to abort. Because I feel that I took a life, it is vital that I know why I did so. I had to step away from my religion for a time, but I tried to remain in constant contact with God. I believe that all things happen for a reason, and I am continuing to discover that reason.

As you move through each aspect of your unique healing process, you are doing the greater work of grieving, which we explore in the following chapter, "Facing Loss." If you are a religious woman, especially one who is actively struggling to overcome the religious conflict you feel over your decision, you deserve to grieve your abortion.

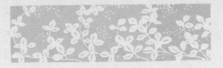

Chapter Seven
Facing Loss

"Everybody must learn this lesson somewhere—that it costs something to be what you are."

—Shirley Abbott
Womenfolks: Growing Up Down South

Grieving enables you to heal the losses born out of your pregnancy and abortion so that, in time, you can move toward a place of emotional peace. As you face and mourn your losses you are able to resolve pain left over from these experiences, but if you dismiss or deny any losses you are apt to prolong your grief.

You might like to believe that the abortion procedure brought an end to the entire experience, but this is not necessarily so. Our psyches will grieve, even if we insist otherwise, and our minds repeatedly kick up old memories and feelings until we face them.

If you feel sad but are afraid to examine your abortion losses or are worried that you will drown in painful emotions, the first exercise in this chapter may help you begin the process of grieving.

Exercise One:

"Endings" and "losses" are a normal part of life. An ending might be a graduation from college or the loss of a relationship. Endings can be forced upon us, as in the death of a loved one, or they can be conscious changes, such as a move to a new place. If you examine your own life history you will surely find several examples of "losses" you have lived through. You may have already grieved some of these losses, while others may linger as unfinished emotional business. Still others may not even be viewed as "losses," but as positive changes in your life.

> Loss is nothing else but change, and change is Nature's delight.
>
> —Marcus Aurelius
> *Meditations*

Whenever there is an ending or transition, even when re- garded as positive, we let go of a part of our life and experience losses. For example, when you completed high school your life may have expanded with new possibilities, but this transition may have meant saying good-bye to special friends and a comfortable routine.

When you had an abortion, you may have chosen to create an ending because you were not prepared to properly care for a child. It may have allowed you to continue on your chosen path, but the decision may have also meant the difficult loss of a pregnancy that a part of you wanted to keep.

Use your journal to address the following:

1. List some of the endings in your life.
2. Consider these questions as you look at your list:

   a. Which of these endings were forced upon you and which did you choose?
   b. What "losses" came out of these endings?
   c. Which of these endings were positive changes but still created losses that were painful for you?
   d. How did you mourn these losses? How and when might they still cause you pain?

Understanding that endings are normal can help you be less fearful of facing losses. Helping you identify and mourn the losses brought about by your pregnancy and its termination is the goal of this chapter.

Recognizing Abortion as a Loss

One of the greatest obstacles between you and your post-abortion grieving may be the lack of cultural and personal recognition that you have suffered a loss. The reasons for this are easy to cite.

> Sorrow is a fruit; God does not allow it to grow on a branch that is too weak to bear it.
>
> —Victor Hugo

First and foremost, we live in a society that rebels against the reality that painful events warrant pain-filled reactions. All we have to do is look around us to find examples of this belief.

How many times have we seen a parent coach a child to stop crying by saying "Big girls [or boys] don't cry." And, every day in professional athletics, television announcers praise players who are "good sports" and who hide their disappointment when they lose a game—no matter what they had at stake. Even in times of terrible anguish, self-restraint is lauded. A stunning example of this occurred in 1963, when the American media hailed Jacqueline Kennedy for not shedding a tear at her own husband's funeral.

These messages erroneously teach us that it is mature to suppress our pain. Reversing these messages is vital if we are to successfully face and mourn our losses. Psychiatrist and author Charles Whitfield reminds us, "When we allow ourselves to feel these painful feelings, and when we share the grief with safe and supportive others, we are able to complete our grief work and thus be free of it."

Women further hesitate to mourn their terminated pregnancies because society does not recognize abortion as a loss. The necessary grieving over a miscarriage has also been thwarted but in a lesser way. Authors and therapists Marie Allen and Shelly Marks speak about this in their research on miscarriage: "We felt that our babies and our losses were not valid and our grief was not justifiable next to babies and losses that were verifiable as 'real.' "

Among many women who have aborted fetuses, this sentiment rings equally true. They have lost something that, in the eyes of many people, never existed. To complicate matters, post-abortion women may question their entitlement to grieve because they chose their loss.

> I know it takes time to heal a painful wound, especially one affecting your heart.
>
> —Edith Mize
> "A Mother Mourns and Grows"
> *Death—The Final Stage of Life,* Kübler-Ross, ed.

Women who support the pro-choice movement may also feel that they have no right to grieve. They may find themselves shrinking from sorrow because they are unwilling to admit that the fetus they let go had meaning to them. Should they feel any emotional or maternal attachment, they might face untenable conflict, especially if they want to believe that this "potential life" was nothing more than discarded tissue.

What such women may have ignored is that the fetus they released can represent normal losses commonly felt by many post-abortion women. Exploring these losses can help you understand the roots of your grief.

Loss of the Fantasy Baby

Reflecting upon one's loss, and even the desire to reclaim what was lost, is a part of grieving familiar to individuals who have suffered the death of a loved one, according to psychologist John Bowlby. From this pain arise persistent thoughts of what life would be like if only "things had been different" and the loss had never happened. For a post-abortion woman, whose loss was her fetus, this process of reflection occasionally gives rise to dreams of the "fantasy baby"— a child she did not choose to have but whom she often fantasizes about.

Persistent thoughts of a fantasy baby are the psyche's way of signaling that there is still grieving to be done. Resisting the urge to reflect upon the meaning of "the baby" prevents closure of the abortion experience.

In finishing dealing with her abortion loss, it is normal for a woman to find herself wondering about the baby she did not have, even to the point of missing the child it would have become. She may feel sorrow over the loss of her "firstborn" if the pregnancy was her first conception or if motherhood was desired but ultimately never realized. She also may feel sorrow if she already had children and now wonders what life would have been like with a larger family.

> Grief should be the instructor of the wise;
> Sorrow is Knowledge.
>
> —Lord Byron
> *Manfred*

If a woman has never come to terms with her decision to abort, she may idealize the baby and imagine how things could have been had she made a different choice. As the fantasy allows her to picture life with that child, she may find herself suffering the pain of her indecision and possible loss. The fantasy may help move her grieving forward as she recalls and reaffirms the reasons why she chose to end her pregnancy.

Pamela, twenty-seven, had her abortion only six months before our interview. She shares her reflections on the fantasy baby:

Things You May Have Lost:

1. your old identity
2. the male partner
3. the baby or the "fantasy baby"
4. a sense of innocence
5. self-esteem
6. motherhood
7. a life vision
8. spirituality
9. body image

I think I've imagined the baby because I have felt so conflicted about this abortion. Had I gotten pregnant in another year, I would have kept it. By then my fiancé and I would be married and settled. I couldn't get it out of my mind. My fiancé said that all these thoughts about the baby were unhealthy, but they seemed important to me.

Pamela told us that, after several months of letting herself "obsess," and three months of work with a psychotherapist, she realized that she had released her fantasy baby through the messages given to her in several dreams:

> Our [women's] bodies are shaped to bear children, and our lives are a working-out of the processes of creation.
>
> —Phyllis McGinley
> "The Honor of Being a Woman"
> *The Province of the Heart*

In the final dream I was walking through a nursery filled with babies crawling on the floor. I walked over to the baby that I knew was mine, and something made me turn around. There was a couple behind me who picked up my baby and walked away. They were so happy to have her. The dream assured me that they were ready for a baby, but I was not. It made me feel more peaceful, as if the baby were going to be safe.

Pamela was fortunate to have a strong connection to her inner life. But with time, work and patience, almost any woman can recognize her loss, experience her grief and resolve her pain.

A woman's chances of lingering too long in fantasy are slight if she recognizes her reasons for aborting. However, if her current life is unsatisfying, the fantasy baby can symbolize a "missed" opportunity and one that she believes would have made her life more "fulfilling." To resolve her loss, she must find value in what she possesses in the present and work toward fulfilling her current goals and dreams.

Lingering in fantasy might also be a means of denying the reality of the loss if a woman believes that the fetus she released was not "potential life," but a real baby. In this case, she might need a formal way to say good-bye to the "real baby" at the heart of her loss. The second step of the following exercise can help you do so.

Exercise Two:

1. If you have found yourself thinking about the fantasy baby, describe these thoughts. What kinds of emotions have you felt?

2. If the fantasy baby has represented the loss of a real baby, it is important to honor the loss of that relationship. You can do so by writing a letter to the baby, even giving the baby a name if you desire. You might tell the baby what its loss has meant to you, and express regrets or guilt you may feel. Remember, you had reasons for your abortion, and it is important that the baby understand what those reasons were.

Loss of the Dream of Motherhood

With every pregnancy comes the potential for motherhood, and with every abortion comes the decision that mothering that particular fetus will be denied. This poignant truth sometimes haunts women in the days after their abortion, regardless of how strongly they believe that their decision to terminate was right.

> The bond between mother and child is the most intimate bond in human experience. In this most primary of human relationships, love, welcome, and receptivity should be present in abundance.
>
> —Christiane Northrup, M.D.
> *Women's Bodies, Women's Wisdom*

While thoughts of the fantasy baby revolve around the identity of the child that was released, thoughts of motherhood involve a woman's relationship with her own identity as a creator of life. Motherhood evokes visions of the family, the drive to nest and settle, and the desire to nurture, protect, teach and love one who is vulnerable and dependent.

The terrible fear that this experience of motherhood will go unrealized is common among women who desire children, whether they have had an abortion or not—but for the still childless post-abortion woman, the fear of losing this dream becomes all too real because, for a time, the dream was nearly reality. Without knowing whether she will ever be pregnant again, her sorrow is heightened. For Amy, the possible death of her dream of motherhood came with her abortion at eighteen:

Motherhood was always in the cards for me from the time I was a little girl. But Lewis was going off to college. Before I discovered I was pregnant, I took him to the airport in our little town. I couldn't walk him in because we were different races and people gossiped like crazy. I remember sitting in the driver's seat and watching him take his suitcases out of the back of the car. I watched him walk away from the car through the rearview mirror. I was sobbing. Then I drove back to my parents' house. Two weeks later I found out I was pregnant. I knew I couldn't have the baby, and I felt sick and awful. I was so scared that I would never have my dream of motherhood come true.

> Emptying my womb became a relief when that "maybe" life was honored, respected, and mourned by the mother I became for an instant but would not stay.
>
> —Anne
> Interview

Twenty-two years passed in Amy's life before she and her husband had a child. During that time, her fear that the dream of motherhood was lost occasionally returned. She went through several difficult relationships, established her career, created deep and rich friendships and saw her life flourish. But she also had another abortion and a painful miscarriage before giving birth to her son.

Echoes of loss may reverberate for post-abortion women, even when they have realized the dream of motherhood. As Beatrice, a mother of two adult children, explains,

I would hope that one does not endlessly mourn the loss of the child that was aborted. How sad that would be. Nevertheless, I have wondered what mothering that child would have been like for me. And because each experience of motherhood has been fulfilling for me, I am certain that this missed opportunity would have been equally rich. It is sad. But not tragic.

The drive to mother, and the loss of the experience, can be life-altering. It means the woman will never know the experience of mothering that child, and sometimes it means she will never explore that unique facet of her female nature.

Exercise Three:

If the loss of motherhood has been painful for you, consider the following questions:

1. If you had other children at the time of your abortion, what did you feel about motherhood then?
2. If you didn't have children at the time, did you worry that the pregnancy you aborted was your last or only chance to become a mother? Do you still worry about that?
3. What does "motherhood" mean to you now? What kinds of feelings does it evoke?

> The memories of long love gather like drifting snow, poignant as the mandarin ducks who float side by side in sleep.
>
> —Lady Murasaki
> *The Tale of Genji*

Recollections of the Man

Oftentimes it seems impossible for a woman to recall her abortion without thinking about the man who impregnated her. With these thoughts may come unanswered questions or feelings of longing. She might wonder how they would have raised that imagined baby and how the baby would have changed their lives. If she is no longer with the man, she might wonder if they would have married or avoided divorce had she decided against aborting.

Sometimes a woman's questioning reveals a sense of loss that is less about the man she knew, and more about her desire to realize a special bond. As Laura describes,

There is a sense of having forged a bond with a man and a baby, a bond that cannot be broken. Soon after my abortion I went to a party and met a woman in her eighth month of pregnancy. I had a sense of loss that was unbelievable. Here was a woman who was secure in these two bonds: the child that would be completely dependent upon her and the man who had created this child with her. They were experiencing a commitment to each other that was secure, like nothing I had in my life.

Other times a woman's feelings of loss are linked to positive recollections of her relationship. As she mourns her abortion, she may think back to memories of that man and the times they shared. Kate, now forty-five, recalls "how dear" her lover was, especially during her abortion:

> Intimacy requires courage because risk is inescapable. We cannot know at the outset how the relationship will affect us.
>
> —Rollo May
> *The Courage to Create*

As much as I loved Anthony, I didn't see us spending our lives together. When I got unexpectedly pregnant at thirty-four and on birth control, he was completely nonjudgmental and fearless. His response enabled me to see that we were in this problem together and that we would solve it together. I think back to that support and feel the loss of what he gave me during that time—really unconditional love and friendship. I can't think of my abortion and not think of him.

Thinking back to the relationship that created your pregnancy is a normal part of post-abortion grieving. If there are losses associated with that relationship, which have never been healed, this is the time to recognize them.

Exercise Four:

1. What was your relationship to the man?
2. What is it now?
3. If it ended, how did it end? Did it relate to the abortion? Did you find ways to feel finished?
4. If you're still together, did a phase of your relationship end? Was it a complicated ending? How has the abortion affected your relationship?

5. If you were (or are) able to talk to that man about your abortion today, what would you say?

Loss and the Female Life Cycle

Feelings of loss over an abortion do not always arise as the experience is occurring, especially if a woman is young and feels that she has ample time to begin a family. Her grief over a terminated pregnancy in her teens and twenties may not surface until she becomes more mature.

> In middle age we are apt to reach the horrifying conclusion that all sorrow, all pain, all passionate regret and loss and bitter disillusionment are self-made.
>
> —Kathleen Norris
> *Hands Full of Living*

When a woman is in her teens or early twenties, she may not view an abortion as the termination of a "potential life." Her immediate goals may be aimed at personal growth, developing her own lifestyle, experimenting with various jobs or attending school. Therefore, her unplanned pregnancy is an obstacle to surmount rather than a missed opportunity for motherhood.

As a woman moves into her thirties and forties, a stronger sense of self often helps her to define her life. She may build a relationship, become a homemaker, clarify career goals and gain financial stability. Concurrently, she may find herself experiencing the influence of hormonal shifts, a heightened appreciation for life and an awareness that her reproductive years are finite. These physical and emotional changes can give way to a reevaluation of where she wants to direct her energies. The prospect of creating a family or making a bigger family are natural concerns.

Sometimes a woman's heightened maturity rekindles memories of a pregnancy she chose to end in younger days. She may find herself unexpectedly struck by new insights and changing priorities. Emily states,

I can answer one thing with certainty; I would not default to the unquestioning decision to abort that I made when I was nineteen.

My life has changed a great deal in twenty years, and I have grown as
a woman.

It is important that a woman not interpret her new insights as
cause to condemn a past decision to abort. If she feels sorrow over the
loss of a fetus, she must remember that the female life cycle dictates
different choices at different stages in a woman's development. The
woman who grieves in her thirties, forties and beyond is
not the same woman who chose an abortion in her teens
or twenties. And, if she compares her current circumstances with those in the past, she may come to a new
appreciation of the decision she made—even if she feels
she could now support and nurture the fetus she released.
Jessica, forty-two, speaks of this awareness:

> Everyone carries
> [grief] alone, his
> own burden, his
> own way.
> —Anne Morrow
> Lindbergh
> *Dearly Beloved*

> I'm sure that if I did get pregnant now, it would be
> very hard to make the decision to have an abortion. Even though I
> haven't had a goal to have a child, my life is rich enough now that a
> child would thrive. Sometimes I feel the loss of not experiencing
> motherhood, but I don't regret the abortion I had at nineteen. And I
> have never made a judgment that I was bad or wrong. It was a
> different time in my life.

Women entering menopause and those whose childbearing
days are long past are also vulnerable to new perspectives. Now in
her mid-forties, Julie, who had her first and only child at thirty-
nine, says,

> I grieve that the option to have another child will not be available to
> me much longer. It makes me revisit my two abortions in a very
> poignant way. I spent all that time getting rid of pregnancies or trying
> to prevent them, and now there won't be any more coming.

When a woman opens herself to a new understanding of her maturing body and its relationship to her psyche, she embraces the reality that the two are inextricably linked.

Exercise Five:

You may relate to some or all of the losses we have described thus far, but there are probably still more losses related to your abortion and individual experience. It is important to identify and face these areas so that you can grieve them at last.

> And when we grieve our losses to completion, we grow.
>
> —Charles L. Whitfield, M.D.
>
> *Healing the Child Within*

1. Make a list of your abortion losses. You can start with the losses we have already mentioned in this chapter. Other areas of abortion loss to consider are

   - the loss of a job or career
   - the loss of your lover
   - the loss of a friend
   - the loss of family support and love
   - the loss of your ability to conceive in the future
   - the loss of a relationship with a Higher Power
   - the loss of your perfect self-image
   - the loss of self-esteem

2. Go back to each item on your list and ask yourself

   a. When did I first realize this loss?
   b. How does this loss make me feel?
   c. How has this loss changed my life?
   d. What would it mean not to feel this loss any longer?

Expressing Your Grief

No two women grieve in precisely the same way. Grieving styles are unique. There is no right way or wrong way to grieve, as long as you validate your emotions without feeling shameful, dumb or silly for doing so.

Some women grieve alone, while others feel the need to share their pain. Some cry silently, others sob and still others barely shed a tear, yet all are fully involved in the process of healing. We asked women, "What is grieving for you?"

"It's expressing sadness. I talk and cry in my car. I yell. I talk to people who aren't there—like my dad, who passed away."

"Grieving is a profound sense of loss. It's about being alone in the universe. It entails a lot of crying; a lot of rebuilding."

> These are the stages of converting our predicament from tragedy to grace, from confusion to insight and wisdom, from agitation to clarity. They are our pilgrimage toward the truth.
>
> —Stephen Levine
> *Who Dies?*

Grieving Is Physical and Psychological

Grieving is a physical and psychological process that allows an individual to adjust to the pain or trauma of a loss. As a woman begins to mourn she will find herself responding in physical ways. Common symptoms are:

crying	shortness of breath
lack of appetite	increased hunger
a lump in the throat	faintness
excessive fatigue	insomnia.

If she tries to deny her loss, she may experience:

stomach distress	colds
anxiety	tension headaches.

Psychologically, normal post-abortion grief is often accompanied by:

depression	irritability
thoughts of the pregnancy	thoughts of the abortion.

In order to avoid succumbing to unnecessary physical distress or chronic emotional pain, it is important that a woman be willing to express and experience her loss.

"I need a lot of cocooning. I need to comfort and console and pamper myself because I feel lost and alone in that place."

"Grieving is acknowledging an experience and allowing myself to sit and talk about it. It's about moving it from an intellectual level to an emotional level."

"My abortion grieving entailed talking with friends and with my husband. I kept journals. I made pictures. I cried."

With permission to experience her emotions and constructive outlets for doing so, a woman is able to weather the highs and lows that grieving may bring. She knows that her feelings are normal, that they are felt by other post-abortion women and that they can be shared if she needs comfort and support.

> Go to your bosom;
> Knock there, and
> ask your heart what
> it doth know.
>
> —Shakespeare
> *Measure for Measure*

When she understands the process of grieving, she may feel even more security—knowing that her natural pain, in all its colors, is there for a purpose and will eventually pass.

The Process of Grieving

Grieving has five stages, as identified by author Dr. Elisabeth Kübler-Ross. They are:

1. denial
2. anger
3. bargaining
4. depression
5. acceptance.

These five stages are experienced as a dynamic process. They do not take you from the first day of your abortion experience to the last in a neat chronology. Instead, the emotions of grief may flow and circulate around your memories and arise as your unconscious demands.

One is likely to feel confused by this process. There may not appear to be any rhyme or reason to the way in which feelings and memories surface and resurface, each demanding attention from new perspectives. Anne relates,

> As I grieved my abortion, certain memories were much easier to resolve than others. One that I struggled with was my relationship with the man I was involved with. That memory was tough. Sometimes I felt sad over it, and then a week later I'd feel mad, and then sad all over again. It felt like I was getting nowhere for the longest time. Eventually I found myself feeling more peaceful. It just kind of happened.

Anger as soon as fed is dead—
'Tis starving makes it fat.

—Emily Dickinson
Poems, Second Series

As you make your way through the work of grieving you may feel lonely at times. You have reentered the places of separation and solitude where you, and you alone, know the distinctive experience of your pregnancy and abortion. If you are familiar with each aspect of the grieving process, you will have a road map to guide you on your journey toward acceptance.

Denial

Denial is a normal first reaction when a loss occurs. Some psychologists believe it serves a temporary and essential function by protecting the psyche from being overwhelmed by a sudden loss or traumatic event. Eventually the psyche becomes strong enough to withstand the pain of the initial experience and denial is no longer necessary.

However, denial can also be a toxic place if a woman chooses to remain there too long in order to fend off, minimize or postpone the natural pain that accompanies her healing process. She may employ these methods to keep from admitting the extent of her grief and pain.

As a post-abortion woman, you might have told yourself some of the following phrases in order to deny the pain of your experience:

- "It's no big deal."
- "It really wasn't that bad."
- "It wasn't a real abortion, it was a routine D & C."
- "It didn't really bother me."
- "I just feel a little depressed sometimes."
- "Lots of positive affirmations will take care of this."
- "It happened years ago."
- "I just need to let it go."

Denial caps off a deep well of feelings and memories—the keys to arriving at final acceptance of your abortion. Rather than diving in and drowning in a stew of emotions, you can best explore denial by slowly sifting through the contents a little at a time. If you have given yourself permission to examine your abortion experience and to face your losses, you may find that the feelings and memories beneath your denial are starting to heal.

> Sorrow was like the wind. It came in gusts.
> —Marjorie Kinnan Rawlings
> *South Moon Under*

Anger

Anger, as we have already seen, is a normal and healthy emotion often felt by women from the moment they discover they are faced with an abortion. As time passes, their anger seeps into different corners of the experience. They are angry for being pregnant and for having to go through an abortion; angry at men who have abandoned them or could never understand the discomfort they were experiencing as women; angry for having to sacrifice a fetus; angry for having to endure the physical discomfort of a pregnancy; angry for having to deal with doctors and clinical staff; angry at God; angry at the culture; angry at their families; and angry for feeling stupid!

As long as you are willing to recognize your anger, define its sources and express the emotion, you will not likely fall prey to internalized rage or dangerous depression. (See chapter 5, "Anger.")

Bargaining

Bargaining is traditionally thought of as the stage in the grieving process when a woman attempts to strike a deal between herself and God, or some other outside force, in order to secure her future safety. In post-abortion terms, some bargains might be: "I promise to use birth control in the future if you make sure I won't ever go through this again," or "I promise to do lots of helpful things for others, if you don't punish me for aborting."

> Rich tears! What power lies in those falling drops.
> —Mary Delarivier Manley
> *The Royal Mischief*

If a woman has found herself striking bargains, she might want to examine her fears: is she afraid of getting pregnant again or of being punished?

Bargaining often becomes a lesson in cause-and-effect as a woman examines what she "should" have done in order to have avoided the whole mess or at least some of her pain. She might tell herself, "If I had only used birth control—then I wouldn't have become pregnant," "If I hadn't been drunk—then I wouldn't have been raped," "If I had gone to see a doctor sooner—then I would have had an easier abortion," "If I hadn't been ovulating—then this wouldn't have happened."

When this cause-and-effect bargaining is done honestly and without self-flagellation, it affords women the opportunity to learn from their experience. For example, a woman who rationalizes "If I had used my diaphragm, then maybe I wouldn't have gotten pregnant" may be more conscientious about birth control in the future. Our lives are not single-episode fairy tales; instead, we have many personal chapters where we have the opportunity to learn and grow from each success and failure.

Constructive bargaining can enable you to go back over the events of your losses and learn from them. It provides a simple way to assess your strengths and weaknesses. With many rocks turned over in this bargaining process, you can gather information about your pregnancy, your abortion and yourself.

Exercise Six:

1. List the bargains you might have made in your grieving process.

2. If you made a bargain with God, were you doing so out of fear? If so, what was that fear? Do you still have that fear?

3. Do you think you should have struck a bargain with yourself in the past? What was the lesson you wanted yourself to learn?

Depression

Depression is a state in which our normally available mental and emotional energy goes underground. When a woman is depressed she may experience sleep disturbances, changes in eating patterns, a lack of sexual interest or a withdrawal from activities and people.

> Give your sorrow all the space and shelter in yourself that is its due. . . .
> —Etty Hillesum
> An Interrupted Life: The Diaries of Etty Hillesum 1941–1943

As children, few of us are taught how to handle normal feelings of depression. Instead, we are told to "buck up" or to "stop feeling sorry for yourself." If we come to suffer a depression, we may not even know how to recognize the symptoms because we are so accustomed to talking ourselves back into pseudo-happiness.

Most women admit to feeling depressed at some time during their abortion experience, but rather than face this normal feeling, they often try to ignore their depression. They may fear that any validation of their pain will throw them into an emotional tailspin. Usually such fear brings the healing process to a halt.

Feelings of ambivalence are normal when it comes time to recall difficult memories, but the desire to halt the process for a while must be kept in check or a woman may never complete her grieving. It is important to remember that the fear of depression is often much greater than any unhappiness depression might bring, and natural depression always comes to an end.

Perhaps the most predictable emotion accompanying depression is the loss of hope. Many women feel that they will never believe in their personal goodness again. They may worry that they will never feel sexually safe or will never conceive a wanted child. They may think that no one could ever truly love them after "what they've done."

This loss of hope dissipates and leaves as women actively release their sadness and examine the reasons for that hopelessness. The process is lonely and there is no exact right or wrong approach but, as long as one is moving through the grieving process, one is on the right track.

Use the following exercise to help you understand and resolve a lack of hope.

> Life is either a daring adventure or nothing.
>
> —Helen Keller
> *Let Us Have Faith*

Exercise Seven:

1. If you are feeling a lack of hope, list the things you are feeling hopeless about regarding your abortion.

2. In regard to each thing on your list, honestly answer each of the following:

    a. Why do you see this as hopeless?

    b. In reality, is this hopeless or do you merely fear that it is?

    c. Can you do anything to restore your hope? What can you do?

    d. How can you make the process less lonely?

3. When was another time you felt hopeless about something that you eventually accepted?

    a. How did you make your transition out of hopelessness?

    b. What thoughts did you have to restore your beliefs?

    c. What behaviors did you engage in to invigorate yourself?

If you experience a prolonged depression or have a history of depression in your family, which frightens you, it is wise to reach out for guidance and counsel from a professional who can help you in your healing process. You can find a qualified counselor through many women's health clinics or your personal physician. Also see pages 74 and 204 for more information.

Acceptance

A woman can eventually accept all her losses, including the loss of her self-esteem, her old self-view, an opportunity, the man and the fetus. Acceptance of multiple factors can come in waves, one at a time, sometimes ebbing but always flowing again.

There is, of course, no precise closure on grieving. Just like when we come across a photo of a long deceased loved one and feel sadness, a post-abortion woman, reconciled to her losses, may still feel tender emotions when something reminds her of her abortion. This is healthy and human. As Deneen shares,

> When I look back to my abortion, I can feel a soft place for the girl I was. I also feel at peace with her decision because without it, my life would be so different. And I like my life.

Emotional strength does not mean the absence of uncomfortable emotions; it does mean the ability to have such feelings and let them transform. Acceptance is simply the strength to face, experience and integrate your losses. Over time, your emotions will become less painful, but they will always inform you about who you are and where you have been.

> It began in mystery, and it will end in mystery, but what a savage and beautiful country lies in between.
>
> —Diane Ackerman
> *A Natural History of the Senses*

Exercise Eight:

1. When individuals feel sad because of old losses, they often need to make special time for themselves and do things to soothe their pain. Here are some things you may want to do when memories about your abortion arise:

   a. Take a hot bubble bath.
   b. Get a good night's sleep.
   c. Play some music you love, even if it makes you cry.
   d. Buy the soft tissues!

    e. Buy flowers for your home.

    f. Buy yourself a present for being courageous.

    g. Have a great meal with a friend and talk.

    h. Write in your journal.

    i. Talk to a loving God.

    j. Attend a positive spiritual service.

2. Add to the above list those things that have restored your sense of well-being at other times in your life.

> Growth itself contains the germ of happiness.
>
> —Pearl Buck
> *To My Daughters,*
> *with Love*

If you continue to struggle with your grief work, look in the appendix of this book to find further readings on the subject of grieving.

The following chapter, "The Process of Healing," offers many additional exercises and suggestions to help you through your abortion recovery. Some of them continue the final stages of grieving, while others address the various perspectives of your recovery in order to help you move into a deeper acceptance of your past abortion.

PART THREE

Acceptance

Chapter Eight
The Process of Healing

"Nothing strengthens the judgment and quickens the conscience like individual responsibility."

—Elizabeth Cady Stanton
"Solitude of Self"

Transformation can bring understanding that is like an internal light-bulb. It can be a slight glimmer eliciting a "Yes, I can just see the light," or an aurora borealis that causes us to gasp in awe. Either way, it marks the process of healing.

When a woman has had an abortion and moved on, she is no longer exactly the same. When we asked the women we interviewed to "Pick words that define yourself," they readily gave many answers. But when we asked them where their abortion fit into their lives, we found that it was often relegated to a "secret place." A secret place is acceptable if you feel no post-abortion pain, but if your abortion has been buried because it remains a source of shame and discomfort, pay special attention to the healing exercises throughout this chapter.

The following exercises are designed to help you learn more about yourself and your abortion, and to continue your process of transformation. As you gather new insights it is important that you admit them to yourself or to a trusted other. Undelivered communication perpetuates pain and loss. Writing, or even sharing with another person, can move the process of healing forward.

John W. James and Frank Cherry, experts on the grieving process, emphasize that individuals carry their own suffering and that they are ultimately responsible for its healing. So, as you pick out and do the exercises in this chapter, talk to yourself . . . and listen.

> There is nothing permanent except change.
>
> —Heraclitus
> Greek philosopher

Exercise One: Awareness of Changes

1. Make a list of the positive changes you have noticed within yourself since your abortion, or since starting this book. Some changes might be

   a. I have more information about my abortion.

   b. I am more aware of my anger.

   c. I realize my abortion allowed me to pursue my goals.

2. After thinking about the changes you have already experienced, think about the changes you hope to see in the future and respond to the following:

   a. *As I heal from my abortion, I will* seem different to myself in these ways. . . .

   b. As I heal from my abortion, other people will also see me as different. They could then say about me, "*Did you notice that . . .*"

EXAMPLE OF HOW THINGS ARE CHANGED:
Lucy answered the above questions this way:

1. *As I heal from my abortion, I will* feel more secure. I will feel more able to speak my mind to others. When I make mistakes, I won't flash back to my abortion. When I look at a baby, I will remember my abortion with just a touch of sadness, not with so much self-criticism.

2. *Did you notice that* Lucy doesn't apologize for things so much anymore? And did you notice that she isn't spending so much extra time at the office? She seems to do more recreational activities lately. She seems more peaceful too.

Exercise Two: Charting Your Life Pathline

Charting a Life Pathline is a clear way to visually recognize the transitional events in your life that have shaped your history and your character.

> Blessed are they that mourn, for they shall be comforted.
>
> —The Beatitudes

Make a line on a piece of paper (you may want to do this in your journal) that marks your life path from the moment you were born to this minute. Your path can be a straight line or an elaborate, squiggly one. Mark a small square on the line for each major milestone in your life, such as: "Graduation–1986," "Moved to Chicago–1993," "Learned to drive–1991." Next, mark an "X" on the line for every significant loss you have experienced, such as: "Abortion–1993," "Divorced–1981," "Grandpa's death–1981."

Here is an example of Trish's Life Pathline:

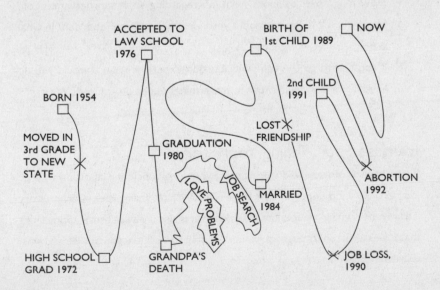

When you finish, sit back with your Life Pathline and notice the life experience you have acquired. Your changes and losses are foundation stones in your character; they help make you the intricate person that you are. Looking at your Life Pathline also allows you to greet the future, to see the life you have yet to live.

Exercise Three: Making Transitions

> How we spend our days is, of course, how we spend our lives.
>
> —Annie Dillard
> *The Writing Life*

Most people can recognize transitional events in their lives but may remain unsure how they managed to get through the difficult times. Answer the following questions to help yourself know more about your personal process.

1. Other than your pregnancy, when have you felt uncomfortable over something you ended in the past?

2. What solutions did you use to help yourself? For example, did you confront someone, did you seek counseling, did you confide in a friend?

3. What do you feel disenchanted about in your life today? People? Goals? Events? Activities?

4. How might past solutions help you regarding your abortion transition?

5. Have you felt differently about your identity since your abortion? In what ways?

6. If you had to go through your abortion experience again, would you do anything differently in order to make things easier on yourself? What?

Exercise Four: Telling Your Story

If you haven't already told the story of your pregnancy and abortion in your journal or to another person, this is the time to do so. Telling your abortion story is a way of "owning" your entire experience. It is also a way of gently appreciating that you have been through an experience that has influenced your life and your character.

Psychotherapists find that when people tell their life stories they often come to value the depth and complexity of themselves. Almost everyone has had the experience of having a marathon conversation with a friend in order to get some problem "off your chest." Even if the friend gives no advice, such storytelling can reduce stress, solve problems, uncover buried emotions and allow you to feel "human."

When we tell our stories we see connections between events. By reexperiencing any upheaval we can identify the specific parts of our past that are healed and those parts that still need attention. This insight can direct us to a problem and allow us to break free from our inner pain. We can choose to heal, lessen the suffering and finally let it go.

> Change is the constant, the signal for rebirth, the egg of the phoenix.
>
> — Christina Baldwin
> *One to One*

Start with the beginning of your relationship with the father, or before, and work your way through to today. Relate the major events and your feelings, then and now. Avoid analysis and your inner "critic."

Exercise Five: Confidence Building

When a woman is in pain, she can easily forget all her talents and positive qualities. Psychotherapist Leslie Eichenbaum recommends a simple exercise that can give you perspective and help rebuild your confidence. As you do this exercise you may be surprised at what you will learn about yourself.

1. Make a list of *ten personal achievements*.
2. Make a list of *ten personal abilities*.
3. Make a list of *ten positive personal qualities*.
4. Imagine that a good friend is introducing you to a third party, in an extremely positive way. Write out what that person would say about you, and when you finish, read the introduction aloud.

EXAMPLES OF CONFIDENCE BUILDING:

After her abortion, Diane felt she needed to remember her strengths. She felt fragile and oversensitive and decided to do this exercise.

1. *Ten Personal Achievements:* Finished school, took a drawing class, had two children, have four very trusted friends, threw a fiftieth wedding anniversary party for my parents, traveled outside the country, helped decorate the lobby at the synagogue, built a fountain in my backyard, gave to a charity, worked to build a healthier marriage.

> When we suppress an emotion, we suppress emotion in general.
>
> —Marie Allen and Shelly Marks
> *Miscarriage: Women Sharing from the Heart*

2. *Ten Personal Abilities:* Can draw, can do kung fu, know a little Spanish, remember important birthdays, am a pretty good cook, can ballroom-dance, know home health remedies, am a good storyteller, am an excellent gift wrapper, can build a campfire.

3. *Ten Positive Personal Qualities:* Loving, caring, funny, smart, clever, creative, intuitive, sensitive, sexy, assertive.

4. *Introduction:*

"I would like to introduce my good friend Diane. She is such a wonderful person. Many times she can intuit what is needed in a situation and then act exactly on what she feels. She is especially intelligent and funny. Not everyone can mix those qualities well, but she certainly can. I appreciate her sensitivity, and I know you will too. She is easy to get to know as she is honest and forthcoming about who she is. And talent! Let me tell you. She does kung fu, draws, travels and camps. With so many positive talents you'd think she was conceited, but it is just the opposite. She is quite humble and loving."

Go ahead and write. Be honest, but don't be modest!

Exercise Six: Things That Need Forgiveness

Forgiving yourself for getting pregnant and having an abortion is essential. It helps you release anger and move forward in your healing. The process of forgiving helps you recognize your humanness.

1. Make a thorough list of the things you have been beating yourself up over. For instance: "I should have used birth control," "I should have been smarter," "I shouldn't have had a drink," or "I should never have had an abortion."
2. Now, write a forgiving statement to yourself for each of the things on your list. For example: "I forgive myself for not using birth control, because I counted the days between my periods wrong."
3. Make a thorough list of the people you are mad at and why.
4. If you feel forgiving (there is no need to force this, as acceptance of your abortion doesn't require forgiving others), make statements of forgiveness for those people on your list you choose to forgive, as you did for yourself in step 2.

> If you think you can, you can. And if you think you can't, you're right.
> —Mary Kay Ash
> *New York Times*

Forgiveness is not always easily reached. You cannot forgive unless you understand what you are forgiving in yourself or another person. Forgiving, as the old expression goes, does not mean forgetting. Remembering the mistakes you made or the wrongs that were done to you helps you remain conscious and aware so that future wrongs happen less and less.

Exercise Seven: Forgiveness Letter to Yourself
Write a letter of forgiveness to yourself. Be fair and be kind.

EXAMPLE OF LETTER OF FORGIVENESS:

Dear [Insert your name],

You are forgiven for having beaten yourself up for five years since your abortion. You are also forgiven for having had an abortion because . . . [Keep on writing until you've said it all].

With love and understanding,

[Insert your name]

Exercise Eight: Saying Good-bye to Your Old Self

As you grow and transform into a healthier woman, old ways of being die. Saying good-bye to your old self helps you to reaffirm how far you have come in your recovery.

1. Get several pieces of paper, a pen, an envelope and a stamp.
2. Write a good-bye letter to your "old self." Include good-byes to old ways of being, thinking and feeling about your abortion. Include things you have learned from having had an unwanted pregnancy and abortion. Include thank-yous for anything gained from your old self.
3. When you have finished, address the envelope to yourself, stamp it and mail it. When it arrives at your home, put it away until you have quiet time to read it. Read it carefully.

> Forgiveness is the act of admitting that we are like other people.
> —Christina Baldwin
> *Life's Companion, Journal Writing as a Spiritual Quest*

EXAMPLE OF SAYING GOOD-BYE TO YOUR OLD SELF:

Marianne took a spiral notebook and pencil, went into her backyard, sat in the grass with her cats and wrote the following good-bye letter:

"Dear Old Marianne:

It is time I let you go. You truly did want an abortion and you truly did not want to have kids, but you also have suffered enough about your loss.

You are so loving toward every living thing, even your cats, that I know that the decision was painful to you. It is okay to think about the fetus, which might have been a child one day, and it is okay to forgive yourself for having such passionate sex you didn't stop to use a condom. I'm saying good-bye to you, though, because you have suffered enough.

I want to tell you that I have learned a lot from you. You have taught me how important every second is in life. You have taught me to be more responsible for my sexuality and my passions. You have helped me understand the sadness that our childhood has caused us. I mourn that, and I know you do too.

I want to thank you for causing me to look deeply within. You quit therapy several times, but after your abortion, you really made a commitment. Thank you for giving me more self-love and care. I will miss you, but it is time for you to go because you have spent enough time going over and over your abortion pain. I want you to let me come forth and celebrate who I am becoming. I love you.

Sincerely,

The New Marianne"

Exercise Nine: Journal Letters

> To err is human, to forgive divine.
> —Alexander Pope
> *The Eternal Now*

Journal letters give you a format to write an imaginary letter to yourself or to someone else in your own journal. It has five specific steps, which are inspired by author John Gray. It is helpful to go step-by-step because the progression can guide you toward deeper and more complete emotions. Each section may be a paragraph or several pages. The sentences begin as follows:

1. I'm angry because . . .
2. I'm guilty because . . .
3. I'm sad because . . .
4. I need you . . .
5. I love you because . . .

Journal letters are especially useful when you find yourself either emotionally "stuck" or so overflowing with emotions that you can't make sense of them. The five steps can guide you to subtle places within. You might address a letter to the fetus, the father, a family member or even yourself.

EXAMPLE OF JOURNAL LETTER:

Susan wrote a journal letter to her married ex-lover. Although she chose to keep it in her journal when it was finished, the process of writing the letter allowed her to honestly face several difficult issues.

"Dear Jerry,

I'm angry because you controlled me with your anger. I'm furious that you were so standoffish that I was terrified to tell you I got pregnant. I'm angry that you are such an idiot. I'm angry that I had to go through the experience alone. I'm angry that you got off scot-free and that you still have a wife and two kids. I'm angry that when I got pregnant, your job wasn't threatened.

> I did not lose myself all at once. I rubbed out my face over the years, washing away my pain, the same way carvings on stone are worn down by water.
>
> —Amy Tan
> *The Joy Luck Club*

I'm guilty because I wasn't strong enough to ask for your help. I feel guilty for being involved with you in the first place. I feel guilty that I got pregnant at all. I feel guilty that it took me so long to learn a lesson.

I'm sad because I lost the opportunity to have a child. I feel very sad that now I don't have you or a baby. I'm sad that I had to make such a hard decision.

I need you to know that I really loved you. I also need you to know that your love wasn't a good love for me. I need you to know that I am okay. I need you to know that I learned a lot being with you. I need to get on with my life and not ever get involved with a married man again. I need my job to continue going well so that I have a good future.

I love you because of the many days we shared. I love you for giving me attention when I felt like dirt. I love you for how creative you are. I love knowing that I am okay without you.

Lovingly,

Susan"

Exercise Ten: The Self Wheel

The Self Wheel is a working blueprint to help you visualize your inner life. Here is an example of Trish's Self Wheel:

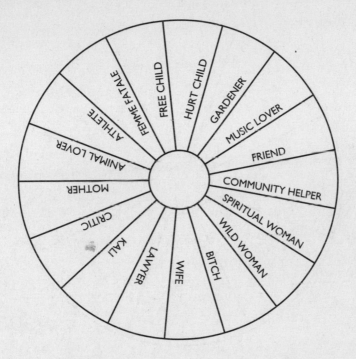

The spokes of the Self Wheel represent the varied aspects of a woman's inner life. Each woman, depending on her character and life situation, has different aspects. Some aspects might be: the daughter, mother, wife, fiancée, adult, animal lover, hurt child, free child, athlete, writer, gardener, musician, teacher, art lover, critic, wild woman, Kali, femme fatale, spiritual woman, worker, lover, caretaker.

Just as liquid needs a container, the contents of a person need a container too—the rim of the wheel represents that container. The place that many women refer to as their "center" or "core" is represented in the wheel by the hub.

On the next page is a blank Self Wheel diagram for you to complete (or you may want to draw this in your journal). Place aspects of your inner life on each "spoke" of the wheel. Add more spokes as you need them. As long as you describe yourself, you can't get the wheel wrong. Put your name above the wheel when you're done.

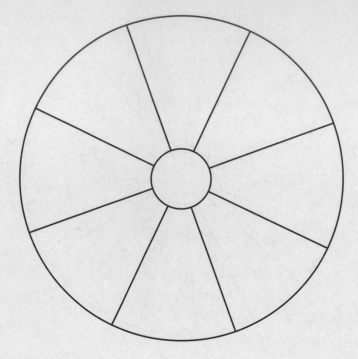

Your awareness of different inner aspects of yourself, or "spokes," allows you the ability to move from spoke to spoke. This is a natural thing that people do, and it is a significant component of being a mature woman. For instance, if a post-abortion woman is stuck in her "critic" spoke and feels significant judgments about her past action, it is essential that she move to another appropriate aspect of her inner life to help her understand the meaning of her abortion. For some women that other spoke may be the "adult," or the "caretaker," or the "spiritual woman" part of themselves.

Remember: each self-aspect contains richness and feeling; the spoke is not a feeling in itself. For example, the "caretaker" may feel many things—strong, patient, frustrated, durable, etc.

Exercise Eleven: Self Wheel Journal Entries

A helpful technique to employ in journal writing is to write from a particular aspect, or "spoke," on your Self Wheel.

1. In your journal, write from one spoke on your Self Wheel.

EXAMPLE OF ONE-SPOKE WRITING:

Lee had "Family Member" on her Self Wheel. She wrote a journal entry from the point of view of that part of herself.

> Family Member speaking: "It is difficult listening to my mom talk on and on about the 'old country.' I must laugh at times because we've been here seventeen years. Yet I too feel callings. I hope to visit there. I can't really remember much, just something about the cold and the airport. I do like to watch my mom when she cooks the fish she learned how to prepare from Grandma. She is silent and calm. In moments like this, I am sad she doesn't know about my abortion. I feel like a traitor, not telling her. Yet, and I cry as I write this, I guess I do not feel like a traitor to her because I protected her by not telling her that I got pregnant in high school. So who's the traitor? Hmm. I don't know. Maybe both of us."

> Why does man accept to live a trivial life? Because of the danger of a full horizon of experience, of course.
>
> —Ernest Becker
> *Denial of Death*

2. In your journal, write letters between two Self Wheel spokes that want or need to talk to each other.

EXAMPLE OF TWO-SPOKE WRITING:

Susan, who chose her new job as a telephone line person over her pregnancy by a married man, wrote a journal letter from her "worker" self to her "lover" self.

> "Dear 'Worker,'
>   I really love and appreciate you because you've taken care of me long after my dreams of Jerry died. You made quite a sacrifice in order to

support me, you worked hard to train for your job and you've purchased us a home. I respect you even if I'm angry you kept me from having my baby. Maybe not angry anymore—just sad. I guess if we were on welfare, or our kid was in day care eight hours a day, I'd be even angrier. I'm just sorry you had to decide so fast. I guess I'm actually thankful too.

Sincerely,

'Lover' "

Who sees the other half of Self, sees Truth.

—Anne Cameron
Daughters of Copper Woman

Susan's inner "worker" wrote back to her own inner "lover."

"Dear 'Lover,'

It's about time I heard from you. You've treated me as if I had the abortion to torture you instead of to support you. You've really pissed me off, and I've wanted to scream at times. Jerry would have been very angry if he knew I was pregnant, and he would have found out for sure—this way it didn't screw up his life with his wife and kids. Having a baby would have really messed up my life too. It hurts us a lot, though, I know. But we're okay. I'm working hard and I love it. I'm also glad Jerry is a thing of the past; I guess I aborted him too. I want you to know that I had to make the decision to abort under time pressure. It was very difficult for me. I'm sorry too. Write more, please.

Yours forever,

'Worker' "

3. Write a "journal letter" between two spokes using the five-step process: anger, guilt, sadness, need and love.

EXAMPLE OF TWO-SPOKE JOURNAL LETTER:
Susan wrote a letter to her "Worker" spoke from her "Lover" spoke using this format. This is a condensed version of her letter:

"Dear 'Worker,'

I am angry with you because your career drive caused me to give up my possible child. I'm angry that you had to keep your job and couldn't be pregnant at the same time.

I am guilty because I feel so ungrateful to you. I feel guilty because you were doing your very best. I feel guilty we aborted.

I am sad because we lost the opportunity to have a child. I'm sad because I love children. I'm sad because I don't have other kids yet.

I need you to know that having an abortion for your career and to take care of us, as a single woman, is appreciated. I need you to know that I know your decision wasn't easy.

I love you because you are strong. I love you because you faced such a difficult period and you are okay now. I love you because you are so sensitive.

Sincerely,

'Lover' "

> Wherever we go, whatever we do, self is the sole subject we study and learn.
>
> —Ralph Waldo Emerson
> *Journals, 1833*

Exercise Twelve: Creating Artwork

Art has long expressed specific or symbolic parts of a person's inner life. Drawing, painting, sculpting, dancing, stringing beads or writing a poem can give form to instinctive heartfelt connections. It is easy to make something artistic that expresses your feelings as long as you don't let your inner "critic" judge you.

EXAMPLE OF CREATING ART: MAKING A COLLAGE

Shanda created a collage by cutting a large rectangle from a cardboard box. She took a stack of old magazines, scissors and glue onto her patio and began to let her imagination roam. She cut out picture after picture of images that represented her abortion experience. She found a theme emerging. Her pictures revealed things that her present life without a child might allow her to accomplish. She found images of traveling and completing her graduate degree. In one small area of the cardboard she also had depictions of girls crying and a tiny cross. She said that little corner represented where the abortion now fit in her life—one corner was enough.

> We are each composed of many parts, each clamoring for expression. We can be held responsible only for the final compromise, not for the wayward impulses of each of the parts.
>
> —Irvin D. Yalom
> *When Nietzsche Wept*

Exercise Thirteen: Creating a Ritual

Rituals are symbolic actions used to honor significant events. We often associate the word "ritual" with a religious act or a time for prayer, but we can find many well-known rituals in our everyday life. We celebrate birthdays with presents and a cake, on New Year's Eve we uncork champagne and sing "Auld Lang Syne," and on Thanksgiving we meet for a traditional meal.

Rituals can also be used to mark important passages in one's personal life or even to set apart special times and events. Many couples have anniversary rituals, and some people see Saturday morning as the time to sleep late, read the paper and have a nice breakfast—these are rituals.

Through the creation of a personal ritual, you can focus on the unique experience of your abortion and honor specific aspects of your healing. You might create a ritual to:

- say good-bye to the fetus;
- say good-bye to an old self-image;
- say good-bye to guilt;
- say good-bye to a lover;
- close the door on disappointment;
- resolve anger;
- reinforce spirituality;
- greet a richer inner self;

- say thanks for what the abortion allowed;
- apologize to the fetus;
- disempower the inner "critic";
- empower the inner "caretaker."

Here are eight elements you might consider when planning a ritual:

1. The Right Space, Time and Light

Rituals can be conducted outside in the backyard, a forest, a meadow, by a lake or any other environment that feels right to you. They can be performed indoors in a private room, such as the den, while the kids are off at school.

The time of day, week or month may be significant to you. Performing a ritual on the anniversary of your abortion, on the date nearest to conception of the fetus, or during your menstrual cycle might carry special meaning.

> One is not born, but rather becomes, a woman.
> —Simone de Beauvoir
> *The Second Sex*

Whether it is night or day, candles can be a powerful element in creating the right ambiance. The actual lighting of candles can also be part of the ritual, and sunlight or moonlight can give further meaning to the setting.

2. Creating a Special Place

Having a special place to set meaningful objects used in a ritual or to focus your attention during a ritual may be important. It could be an elaborately embroidered cloth spread upon a table, a scarf on an upside-down cardboard box, or a palm frond placed upon the ground. Some women like to call this space their "altar."

3. Special Clothing

Just as a bride wears a white dress, donning special clothing can affect your psyche. A favorite scarf or blouse might induce specific feelings and put you in the right mental state for your ritual.

4. Music

Music can be incorporated into a ritual. It can be prerecorded or created on the spot. Many women have meaningful songs that help move their attention into their hearts. Other women make their own sounds by humming a song, playing a favorite musical instrument, shaking a gourd or beating a drum.

5. Readings and Recitations

Art is a form of catharsis.

—Dorothy Parker

Poems, lyrics, journal entries and passages from beloved books can enhance ritual healing. You can read silently or aloud. Spontaneous words can also free your feelings and thoughts.

6. Special Objects

A favorite rock, a vase, a necklace, a feather or a shell are all special objects when they have personal significance to you. Some women also incorporate artwork or photographs.

7. Fragrances and Flowers

Incense, oils, spices and perfumes contribute to a ritual through the power of their aroma. Flowers not only offer a sweet smell—they are also beautiful. Specific flowers and scents may be chosen for their significance to you.

8. Drinks and Food

A special drink, such as spring water, fruit nectar or sweet wine, can amplify or sanctify a ritual. Foods such as nuts and fruits can be placed in a favorite dish and eaten during the ritual.

EXAMPLES OF RITUALS:

Example A—In Japan, many women and men practice a ritual called *mizuko kuyo*, meaning an offering to a "water-child." Stones, representing the guardians of unborn children, are placed within a shrine. Women and men come to pour a ladle of water over the stones in an act of ritual cleansing meant to honor the fetus and bring peace to the mothers and fathers.

Diane, who had an abortion but felt the lack of cultural traditions to acknowledge it, tells us,

> Henry and I were in Japan, and one of the places we were taken to was a Shrine for Unborn Children. It was very powerful to walk through this place. It was the first time I'd thought of my abortion in years. There were monuments, over and over again, to these unborn children and also small stones, like headstones, placed here and there. There was a little altar with a bamboo ladle. You could pour the water on top of a headstone. We performed the ritual. It was very purifying.

> The preparation for the ritual *is* the ritual.
>
> —Kate Green
> *Shattered Moon*

Example B—After Jessica's abortion she and her boyfriend, Alan, traveled to France. While in Paris they visited the Museum of Man, where they saw jars of preserved fetuses. Jessica tells us,

> The experience was surprisingly upsetting, and I knew that there was more to my healing than I'd bargained for. Alan did not want to discuss his feelings, so I had to do something alone. One afternoon, after we returned to the U.S., I set up a small "altar" in my room when my parents weren't home. I lit candles and burned incense. I sang a song about a lost gypsy that I always liked and said good-bye to what I'd always called the "tissue." By the end, I was both sad and released. The ritual helped me so much that several years later, when I lost my brother, I did something very similar to say good-bye to him too.

Example C—Sharon and Richard went into psychotherapy after the termination of a Down's syndrome fetus. Unable to find solace, they decided that they would plant a tree for their lost child. Richard, a landscape designer, felt this would have particularly rich meaning for him. Sharon explains,

> After the abortion, Richard and I and our two-year-old son went to visit my father and his wife. We wanted to plant a tree for the baby

we'd lost, but I wanted to make sure we planted it somewhere where it would be safe. I didn't want it to be cut down some day. We decided on the family farm because we knew the farm would always be there.

Richard bought two trees, one pink and one white flowering dogwood. We planted two trees because I wanted one to be for the lost baby and one for our son. I felt that one tree would be there to protect the other tree.

> Life shrinks or expands in proportion to one's courage.
> —Anaïs Nin

We didn't have anything written because it felt too hard to do. After we put the trees in the ground, my husband had things he wanted to say; he's wonderful with words. It was beautiful. We both cried. My son was there and my parents too. We gave each other hugs, and as I cried my stepmother told me, "Let it out. Just let it all out." She said that when the first blooms came off the tree, she would send them to us.

Rituals such as those performed by Diane, Henry, Jessica, Sharon and Richard can mark a specific loss, decision, change or sacrifice. An abortion can be recognized and honored as one of the many changes we make in life.

If you desire to perform more than one ritual, do so. Most women choose to engage in a private ritual, but you may want to share it with a close friend, family member or spouse.

Exercise Fourteen: Quiet Moments, Meditation and Prayer

Quiet moments can be a means to commune with the spiritual or a deep place inside yourself.

These moments, or meditations, can be simple or formal. You can take a blanket to the woods, sit beneath a canopy of trees and watch birds and squirrels until you feel a sense of calm. You may have a personal word, or mantra, that you repeat until you feel the beating of your own heart and hear inner voices of reassurance and acceptance. Or you may breathe deeply many times while looking at a flower or a sunset.

You can contemplate the meaning of your abortion experience, silently speak to yourself about the time you had it, quietly converse with the fetus you released, or address your Higher Power. You might recite well-known religious prayers or you might write your own. The purpose is to put your abortion experience in a larger context.

In meditation, you may recognize aspects of yourself that are either consuming too much of your attention or are being overlooked. Is your inner "critic" totally forgetting that you chose an abortion to ensure that you would have enough money to feed your other children, or because you were sixteen years old, or because you couldn't tolerate the social stigma of a pregnancy out of wedlock or because you would have lost your job? Listen to the inner voices through meditation and hear which is the loudest and why. Later, you might go back and address the irate and errant voices through a journal letter.

> Health is not a condition of matter, but of Mind.
> —Mary Baker Eddy
> *Science and Health*

Exercise Fifteen: Reclaiming Your Body

Consider ways that you may have cut yourself off from your body since your abortion. Sometimes getting in touch with feelings through the body can be a very strong experience. If at any time during this exercise you feel overwhelmed, stop. Take a walk. Wait to do the exercise at a time you can be with a professional counselor or therapeutic bodyworker.

Lie on a bed or couch and simply be aware of your entire body. Begin by focusing attention on your toes and work your way up to the top of your head. Note any tension or physical discomfort. Contract your muscles in each of these areas and then, with a big exhale, let the tension drop away. After five minutes, pick up your journal and address the following questions:

1. Since your abortion, how has your body been different?
2. Is there a part of your body that has caused you the most concern?
3. Have you neglected to take care of your body since your abortion?
4. What things have you done to tend to your body?
5. What things would you like to do more often?
6. What part of your body makes you cry?

Whether we are weaving tissue in the womb or pictures in the imagination, we create out of our bodies.

—Meinrad Craighead
The Mother's Songs:
Images of God the Mother

Alternative Healing Avenues

If you desire, you can reach outside your own journal, family and circle of friends for professional therapeutic help. Individual psychotherapy with a trusted therapist has helped women, as have couples' therapy and group therapy. It is essential that you find and test the counselor or leader of such therapy in order to ascertain any bias or prejudice. A positive therapeutic experience fosters authentic self-knowledge and acceptance; it does not condemn or induce shame.

Many women recognize that they viscerally feel guilt, humiliation or anger. Sometimes these women have chosen hypnosis, breath work or therapeutic bodywork. In some parts of the country these health care disciplines have become very sophisticated. Women have told us that by identifying where they are holding tension and pent-up feelings in their muscles, they have been able to let go of the hurt—even if it meant crying endlessly session after session for a month.

The Twelve-Step Programs (Alcoholics Anonymous, Al-Anon, Codependents Anonymous, Overeaters Anonymous, etc.) have guided millions of people to their personal understanding of a Higher Power without shame. Personal insights gained in the Twelve-Step Programs may be helpful in aspects of abortion resolution too.

Transformation Is an Ongoing Process

In our interview with Deneen, we asked her if there was anything she might want to share with other women who have had abortions. She says,

> If you haven't looked at your feelings about your abortion, there are probably a lot of other things you haven't looked at too.

Deneen's advice reminds us that transformation occurs in many areas of our lives and that it is an ever evolving process. Just when we think we've arrived at wholeness, we learn something new about ourselves.

Chapter Nine
Acceptance

"I am never afraid of what I know."
—Anna Sewell
Black Beauty

With post-abortion acceptance under way you may have already begun to identify and understand the sources of your discomfort, to nurture yourself through residual feelings and to confront internal voices should they try to judge, shame or punish you for your past action. If old feelings arise, you will be more and more able to tell yourself, "I know what this is. I know where this is coming from. I can work through this."

As you continue your healing, remember that acceptance is an ongoing process in which old wounds are increasingly understood, learned from, lessened and dealt with from a healthier place. Acceptance does not require that you feel completely resolved about each and every aspect of your experience.

Acceptance of your abortion does not mean you will never think back to the event again. You may experience occasional sad memories as you recall your abortion in the years to come. These subtle emotions can be a blessing in disguise. They remind you to recognize the steps you took in order to become the woman you are today, and they remind you that life is filled with a broad array of experiences.

Your grieving may be complete when you can say, "Yes, I had an abortion. I didn't want to have this experience in my life, but I did. I have learned more about life and myself. I am more comfortable with my emotions and less surprised by undesirable events because they are a normal part of life."

As long as your life continues, it will be challenged by difficult experiences that will offer you opportunities for growth.

> But she also knew she was being confronted with the meaning of her own existence and her freedom to choose between life and creativity or her capacity for self-destruction.
>
> —Linda Schierse Leonard
> *Witness to the Fire*

Accepting Change Means Growing

Accepting and growing from change is the core of well-being and health. Just as it is necessary to let old physical images transform in order to accept life as it presents itself, it is also necessary that a woman let old self-concepts change in order to grow emotionally. The woman who resists accepting her past

Acceptance Can Be Found for Many Things:

- Accept yourself for having an abortion.
- Accept the reasons you made the choice at the time.
- Accept that you may wish that you had handled aspects of the situation differently.
- Accept your losses accompanying the experience.
- Accept the meaning of your abortion in your life.
- Accept the changes made to your self-knowledge.
- Accept the growth steps you've taken.

abortion or the woman who regrets her choice and is unable to grow from the reality that life brings hardships, may find herself stuck with an immature concept of what it means to be an adult.

Accepting that you made the choice to end a pregnancy means that you are acknowledging your ability to make life-altering decisions for yourself—even when those decisions create emotional unrest, cause you to question yourself or are controversial.

Accepting that you made the choice to end a pregnancy means that you have released the childish notion that everyone passes through life without adversity.

> Courage is the price that Life exacts for granting peace.
>
> —Amelia Earhart
> *Courage*

Accepting that you made the choice to end a pregnancy means that you are accepting yourself as a woman who is living with ever evolving expectations of yourself and of what your life might bring, rather than impossibly rigid standards of what your self-image and your life should have been like. Psychotherapist Marion Woodman reminds us, "Perfection is defeat . . . perfection belongs to the gods; completeness or wholeness is the most a human being can hope for."

The post-abortion woman who develops her authentic individuality is not a naive child resisting the responsibilities of womanhood: she is a woman well aware of her world and the complexity of living.

Exercise One:

Write a letter to yourself about your acceptance. Tell yourself, as you would tell a friend going through the same experience, the following:

- all the reasons why it is important that you accept who you are—a woman who has had an abortion
- that you know this is not something that you wanted to have happen
- what you might have wanted to do differently, and what you might have done just right

- what you lost and what you gained
- that this has been a painful but powerful time of learning and that you are
  growing.

Acceptance Balanced against Cultural Change

Even when a post-abortion woman has truly accepted that change is normal and that it can be an opportunity for her personal growth, she realizes that the culture she lives in is fraught with controversy and confusion around women's reproductive rights. Although history shows that women have always induced abortions, accepting a past abortion may be especially challenging for a woman at this time of cultural change.

> I love my past. I love my present. I'm not ashamed of what I've had, and I'm not sad because I have it no longer.
>
> —Colette
> *The Last of Cheri*

Our culture has experienced great swings about the status of women. Women have sought equal rights, yet have seen the defeat of the Equal Rights Amendment. They have made strides in the workplace, yet still earn far less money than their male peers. Abortion has been legalized in the United States, yet many women fear character assault and possibly even physical assault should people find out.

It is a challenging world for women, and if they are seeking an external black-and-white "truth" about their abortion, they will come up empty handed; there is no one truth to be had. Nevertheless, some individuals and groups insist that the world consists of clear dualities: dominators and victims, predators and prey, and right and wrong, with no room for a middle ground, multiplicity or exceptions.

These extreme ways of thinking are dangerous when they sneak into a woman's psyche unexamined. When these standards are internalized as the only truth, the woman may feel plagued with judgments and never reach genuine acceptance. Even worse, if she looks outside of herself for acceptance from an authority figure who will only help her if she admits she made a "mistake" by terminating a fetus, she may find a false absolution because it is not her own. It also may be false because she may not believe her abortion was a mistake; instead, it was an experience that left her perplexed, confused and searching for its meaning in her life.

Instead of adopting an external cut-and-dried "truth," the healthy woman must figure out what is psychologically best for her. Responsibility for her post-abortion healing rests solely in her personal values and standards—not society's. If her values genuinely match society's, then good! She will find lots of external support. But if they do not, giving over to cultural beliefs will only leave her feeling like a fake and just as ill at ease about her past abortion as before.

Maya Angelou, America's poet laureate, has written: "The woman who survives intact and happy must be at once tender and tough. She must have convinced herself . . . that she, her values, and her choices are important."

In pursuit of being "tough," a woman must address society's out-of-date definitions, which limit her identity to being solely nurturing, passive, good and cooperative. Healthy female maturity demands that she broaden these confining definitions and realize how expansive her personality truly is. Only then will she know that allowing her needs to be met, even though they may be complex or controversial, is a positive attribute.

> Yes, and I long for one thing more: to learn how to listen to the delicate vibrations of my soul, to be incorruptibly true to myself and fair to others, to find in this way the right measure of my own worth.
>
> —Karen Horney
> *An Awakening Spirit*

To do this, a woman must continually recommit herself to a path of growth and healing. As author Madeleine L'Engle has written, "My job is to live fully as a woman, enjoying the whole of myself and my place in the universe." A woman must lead a conscious life, sifting through the beliefs she has held, assessing which ones are right for her and tossing out those that do not serve her uniqueness. By being courageous in thought and genuine in feeling, she can come to accept herself, her needs and her choices.

When a woman embraces her inner multiplicity, she begins to see the world from a broader perspective and greets her life in a new light. She is neither a perpetrator, who did an unforgivable thing by terminating a pregnancy, nor an emotional hostage to external ideas telling her how she "should" be.

In speaking about her acceptance, Melanie tells us,

> For me, life is a difficult journey—it is not easy and It Is not meant to be easy. I think that with the mentality that it is supposed to be easy, a person sets herself up for victimhood. The art form, I suppose, is to expect and recognize difficulty, and to do it with welcoming arms—not with bitterness. At an early age I lost friends and classmates to the Vietnam War. There have been many losses and hardships since. And there have been joys and rewards too. My abortion is one of the painful things that has happened in my life. Ha! I realize that I didn't just say that it "happened TO me." I'm glad. Things happen—it is a challenge to embrace it all and to approach the world with soul. My soul, your soul and the world's soul.

> Nature never repeats herself, and the possibilities of one human soul will never be found in another.
> —Elizabeth Cady Stanton
> "Solitude of Self"

When Acceptance Arrives

Acceptance does not come simply because an individual is tired of feeling pain. It is a process of subtle revelations about her life and the world she inhabits. Many women we spoke with shared their personal transitions to acceptance.

For Marianne, who had her abortion at twenty-one, the dilemma of accepting herself as a childless woman hindered her resolve for several years. As she matured into her thirties, she realized that the thought of actually parenting a child was not something she truly desired. Marianne explains that her husband's realization that he felt the same way increased her solace and acceptance:

> We watch our niece occasionally on weekends. We've come to realize that neither of us likes the process of parenting for more than

forty-eight hours at a time. So, our closure is, "Boy, we did make the right decision." It was a sad decision, but for us, realistically, it was the right decision.

Maggie and Roger already had a child when they chose to terminate an unplanned pregnancy. Maggie worked part-time and Roger was unemployed. Together, they decided that an additional child would be more than they could handle. Roger says,

> With our growing awareness that womanly strengths have been bent to the needs and ends of others, we have turned at last to-ward delineating, affirming and ex-pressing the self.
> —Emily Hancock
> *The Girl Within*

I feel good that the abortion wasn't wasted. We didn't have the abortion and then blow off all the work that had to be done. It is an act of self-preservation that can be argued. Growth came at great expense. All I know is that I felt really bad, but that this was necessary for Maggie and me to keep our family together. The abortion was a signal that life asks us to make choices and that you can't satisfy everybody and everything. It was an important lesson. It feels like it was one of those tough decisions that life tosses us. We're just not going to come out of life squeaky clean.

Cloe describes her acceptance in a reflective manner with a sense of completion:

I think that acceptance, for me, came with knowing that I just wasn't ready to have a child at twenty-three, and it was okay to let go of the little being growing inside. It was my decision. So be it. I now have children whom I wanted, whom I love and whom I was ready for.

Lee's acceptance came six years after her abortion. Through therapy and a process of journaling and journal letter writing, she came to terms with the young woman who, at seventeen years of age, chose to have an abortion:

Acceptance came late. Considering what I knew about myself and about life when I got pregnant, I really did everything I could. The twenty-four-year-old me was guilty, but the high school junior wasn't—she had done her best. I learned to appreciate that the seventeen-year-old was a damn brave kid. I am in no way proud of my abortion. I wish it hadn't happened. I am sad to have had this in my life. But I am also relieved to know that I am not a weak person.

Jenny's acceptance of her abortion at the age of thirty-two arrived without undue struggle. She shares,

> Life was meant to be lived and curiosity must be kept alive. One must never, for whatever reason, turn his back on life.
>
> —Eleanor Roosevelt
> *Autobiography of Eleanor Roosevelt*

How did I accept my abortion? That's a great question. Well, first of all, I wasn't married and I didn't want to be a single mother, even with a pretty good career. Second, as a black woman who had a white lover, I just didn't think that I wanted to have an interracial child. I think that can make life hard on a child, the sense of not really belonging, and life is so tough anyway. I guess the acceptance was that I knew why I was aborting and my reasons were so clear. I felt lousy about the whole thing, but I still felt that it was right.

Trish tells us,

I find myself evolving, personally. I find myself more open and questioning about my character. And the mystery of life interests me.

Laura relates,

I have made every effort to honor my vow to myself that I would not create another life that had to be destroyed, but that does not in any way affect my sense that abortion was the right thing for me to do. . . .

Anne shares,

Around the time of my abortion a dear friend sent me a poem. Through my days of healing I read and reread it. I was reminded that life is a state of unexpected change, and the best one can do is to be aware of one's life as it happens, to grow and know that as life keeps changing so must we.

> Blessed sister, holy mother, spirit of the fountain, spirit of the garden, Suffer us not to mock ourselves with falsehood.
> —T. S. Eliot
> Ash Wednesday

Many women have arrived at acceptance in their own ways and at different paces: through therapy, quiet time, writing their thoughts, crying and expressing relief over days, weeks, months and years. All of them came to realize that their decisions were not made in a vacuum but as a result of addressing the events and circumstances in their lives. By deeply exploring and valuing their decision, they were able to achieve acceptance.

Maintain Your Insights and Keep Them Growing

Your insights need help to be sustained, because it is not uncommon for people to lose hard-won "Aha's!"

There is a Zen saying, "To clean up the universe, clean up your own backyard." Anyone who has ever tended a garden knows the labor required to achieve healthy, beautiful plants. Getting the flowers to grow, holding the weeds at bay, knowing what needs sun and what needs shade, understanding which are the friendly bugs and which are the nasty ones—all of this demands study, patience and sweat.

In order to tend to your life—your universe—you need to become a gardener to your inner world. Like gardening, this work asks for patience and sweat. And, like gardening, new beginnings are usually small and unimpressive. It doesn't matter how quickly the results come. It only matters that you are in the process of doing the work—in the process of living a healthier life.

Exercise Two:

Here are some things you can do to reinforce what you are discovering:

1. Reread the exercises, feelings and thoughts you've recorded in your journal and remember all that you have been through and all that you have learned.

> Action should culminate in wisdom.
> —*Bhagavad Gita*

2. Anniversary dates are a normal time to be upset. Don't expect to have a very happy day. Make plans ahead of time. Write in your journal about the past date. Plan enjoyable activities, perform a ritual, be with a friend who understands you.

3. Approach your sex life with patience if you've had trouble there. Use birth control that you have confidence in.

4. Get rid of reminders. If your doctor, clinic, clothes or an activity brings up too much pain, don't be afraid to make changes.

5. Desensitize yourself to those things you cannot change. If a song that hurts you keeps popping up on the radio, buy it and listen to it many times while doing an enjoyable activity. If a cologne or a particular flower triggers memories, use it many times in positive settings. The hurtful associations will diminish.

6. Collect inspirational poems and sayings, or write your own. Put them in conspicuous places or read them when you need support.

7. Be a resource for other women going through abortion healing. Helping them can allow your grieving to finish and your new perspective to take hold.

Add your personal ideas to the ones we have given you.

8. _____

9. _____

10. _____

Go back and do the exercises in this book again and again, if you need to. Recognize which chapters sting the most and which give you the most solace. Sit with them for a while. Pay attention to your intuition. If you become aware of other issues in your life that need attention, take care of them too. Take care of yourself.

Reclaim and master the complexity of being a woman. And know that it is perfectly acceptable to feel responsible to better your life and to heal your abortion—you are responsible!

Selected

Bibliography

Adler, Nancy E., Henry P. David, Brenda N. Major, Susan H. Roth, Nancy F. Russo and Gail E. Wyatt. "Psychological Responses After Abortion." Science. Vol. 248. pp. 1–116. 1990.

Adler, Nancy E., et al. "Psychological Factors in Abortion: A Review." American Psychologist. Vol. 47, No. 10, pp. 1194–1204. October 1992.

Allen, Marie, Ph.D., and Shelly Marks, M.S. *Miscarriage: Women Sharing from the Heart*. New York: John Wiley & Sons Inc. 1993.

Angelou, Maya. *Wouldn't Take Nothing for My Journey Now*. New York: Random House. 1993.

Benvenuti, P., et al. "Abortion and the Man; Psychological and Psychopathological Manifestations in the Face of Lost Fatherhood." *Riv Patol. Nerv. Ment.*, Italy. Nov.–Dec. 1978, 104(6), pp. 255–68.

Bonavoglia, Angela. *The Choices We Made: 25 Women and Men Speak Out About Abortion*. New York: Random House. 1991.

The Boston Women's Health Book Collective. *The New Our Bodies, Ourselves*. New York: Simon & Schuster. 1984.

Bowlby, John. *Loss*. New York: Basic Books. 1980.

Bradshaw, John. *Healing the Shame That Binds You*. Deerfield Beach, Fla.: Health Communications, Inc. 1988.

Carcy, Peter. "A Small Memorial: To the Children the Author Tried to Forget." The New Yorker. Sept. 25, 1995.

Congleton, G. Kam and Lawrence G. Calhoun. "Post-Abortion Perceptions: A Comparison of Self-Identified Distressed and Nondistressed Populations." The International Journal of Social Psychiatry. Vol. 39, No. 4. pp. 255–265. Winter 1993.

de Castillejo, Irene Claremont. *Knowing Woman: A Feminine Psychology.* New York: Harper & Row. 1973.

Erikson, Erik H. *Identity and the Life Cycle.* New York: W.W. Norton & Company. 1980.

French, Marilyn. *The War Against Women.* New York: Ballantine Books. 1992.

Friday, Nancy. *My Mother/My Self.* New York: Delacorte Press. 1977.

Gilligan, Carol. *In a Different Voice: Psychological Theory and Women's Development.* Cambridge, Mass.: Harvard University Press. 1982.

Gimbutas, Marija, ed. *The Civilization of the Goddess: The World of Old Europe.* New York: HarperCollins. 1991.

Hancock, Emily. *The Girl Within: Recapture the Childhood Self, the Key to Female Identity.* New York: E.P. Dutton & Company. 1989.

Kübler-Ross, Elisabeth. *On Death and Dying.* London: Collier-Macmillan, Ltd. 1969.

LaFleur, Williman. "Abortion Practices in Japan and What They Can Teach the West." TRICYCLE: The Buddhist Review. pp. 41–44. Summer 1995.

Lerner, Harriet Goldhor, Ph.D. *The Dance of Anger.* New York: Harper & Row. 1985.

Levine, Stephen. *Who Dies? An Investigation of Conscious Living and Conscious Dying.* New York: Doubleday. 1982.

Lowinsky, Naomi Ruth, Ph.D. *The Motherline: Every Woman's Journey to Find Her Female Roots.* New York: Jeremy P. Tarcher, Inc. 1992.

May, Rollo, Ph.D. *Man's Search for Himself.* New York: W.W. Norton & Company. 1953.

Miller, Jean Baker, M.D. *Toward a New Psychology of Women.* Boston: Beacon Press. 1976.

Murdock, Maureen. *The Heroine's Journey.* Boston: Shambhala. 1990.

Reddy, Maureen T., Martha Roth and Amy Sheldon, eds. *Mother Journeys: Feminists Write about Mothering.* Minneapolis: Spinsters Ink. 1994.

Rosenfeld, Jo Ann and Tom Townsend. "Doesn't Everyone Grieve in the Abortion Choice?" The Journal of Clinical Ethics. Vol. 4, No. 2. pp. 175–177. Summer 1993.

Rosenfeld, Jo Ann, M.D. "Emotional Responses to Therapeutic Abortion." American Family Physician. Vol. 45, No. 1. pp. 137–142. January 1992.

Sheehy, Gail. *Passages: Predictable Crises of Adult Life.* New York: E.P. Dutton & Company. 1974.

Steinberg, Terry Nicole. "Abortion Counseling: To Benefit Maternal Health." American Journal of Law and Medicine. Vol. 15, No. 4. pp. 483–517. 1989.

Viorst, Judith. *Necessary Losses: The Loves, Illusions, Dependencies and Impossible Expectations That All of Us Have to Give Up in Order to Grow.* New York: Ballantine Books. 1986.

Appendix I
Feelings List

abandoned
abused
accepted
affection
afraid
aggravated
alone
amazed
amused
angry
annoyed
anxious
appreciative
ashamed
awful
awkward

baffled
belittled
belligerent

bitter
bored

calm
capable
cheapened
cheerful
competent
confident
confused
content
criticized
crushed

defeated
dejected
demoralized
depressed
despair
despised

discouraged
disliked
dissatisfied
distrustful
doubtful

ecstatic
embarrassed
empty
enraged
envious
excited
excluded
exhausted
exposed

fantastic
fearful
fine
foolish

frantic
friendly
frightened
furious

glad
good
grateful
great
guilty

happy
hateful
hatred
helpful
helpless
hesitant
hopeless
humble
humiliated
hurt

ignored
imprisoned
inadequate
incompetent
inept
inferior
insecure
intimidated
irritated

jealous
jilted
joyful

lonely
longing
loved
loving

mad
maligned
miserable
misunderstood

needed
neglected
nervous

oppressed
optimistic
ostracized
outraged
overwhelmed

panicky
passionate
pleased
powerless
pressured
puzzled

regretful
rejected
relaxed
relieved
resentful
ridiculed
ridiculous
rotten

sad
satisfied
scared
selfish
serene
shocked
skeptical
spiteful
startled
surprised
suspicious

tense
terrible
threatened
thrilled
trusting

uncertain
uncomfortable
uncooperative
understood
unimportant
unloved
unsatisfied
unsure
upset

wanted
warmhearted
worried
worthless
worthy

Appendix 2

Resources: Reading List

Abortion

Bonavoglia, Angela. *The Choices We Made: 25 Women and Men Speak Out About Abortion.* New York: Random House. 1991.

Tribe, Laurence H. *The Clash of Absolutes.* New York: W.W. Norton & Company. 1992.

Alcoholism

Black, Claudia, Ph.D., M.S.W. *It Will Never Happen to Me.* Denver: MAC Publishing. 1981.

———. *Repeat After Me.* Denver: MAC Publishing. 1985.

Gravitz, Herbert L. and Julie D. Bowden. *Recovery: A Guide for Adult Children of Alcoholics.* New York: Fireside. 1985.

Leonard, Linda Schierse. *Witness to the Fire: Creativity and the Veil of Addiction.* Boston: Shambhala. 1990.

Anger

Lerner, Harriet Goldhor, Ph.D. *The Dance of Anger.* New York: Harper & Row. 1985.

Creative Expression

Cameron, Julia and Mark Bryan. *The Artist's Way: A Spiritual Path to Higher Creativity.* New York: G.P. Putnam's Sons. 1992.

Eating Disorders

Chernin, Kim. *The Hungry Self: Women, Eating & Identity.* New York: Random House. 1985.

Kano, Susan. *Making Peace with Food: Freeing Yourself from the Diet/Weight Obsession.* New York: Harper & Row. 1989.

Roth, Geneen. *Feeding the Hungry Heart: The Experience of Compulsive Eating.* New York: New American Library. 1982.

Woodman, Marion. *Addiction to Perfection.* Toronto: Inner City. 1982.

Family Healing

Bradshaw, John. *Bradshaw on: The Family.* Deerfield Beach, Fla.: Health Communications, Inc. 1988.

Miller, Alice. *The Drama of the Gifted Child.* New York: Basic Books. 1981.

Whitfield, Charles L., M.D. *Healing the Child Within: Discovery and Recovery for Adult Children of Dysfunctional Families.* Deerfield Beach, Fla.: Health Communications, Inc. 1987.

Grief

Kübler-Ross, Elisabeth. *On Death and Dying.* London: Collier-Macmillan Ltd. 1969.

Kushner, Harold. *When Bad Things Happen to Good People.* New York: Schocken Books. 1981.

Levine, Stephen. *Who Dies? An Investigation of Conscious Living and Conscious Dying.* New York: Doubleday. 1982.

Inspirational/Spiritual

Angelou, Maya. *Wouldn't Take Nothing for My Journey Now.* New York: Random House. 1993.

Canfield, Jack and Mark Victor Hansen. *Chicken Soup for the Soul*. Deerfield Beach, Fla.: Health Communications, Inc. 1993.

Fields, Rick, Peggy Taylor, Rex Weyler and Rick Ingrasci. *Chop Wood, Carry Water: A Guide to Finding Spiritual Fulfillment in Everyday Life*. Los Angeles: Jeremy P. Tarcher, Inc. 1984.

Lindbergh, Anne Morrow. *Gift from the Sea*. New York: Random House. 1978.

Morgan, Marlo. *Mutant Message Down Under*. New York: HarperPerennial, 1995.

Sargent, Claudia Karabaic. *An Awakening Spirit: Meditations by Women for Women*. Peg Streep, ed. New York: Viking Penguin. 1993.

Stein, Diane. *Casting the Circle: A Woman's Book of Ritual*. Freedom, Calif.: The Crossing Press. 1990.

Men's Healing

Absher, Tom. *Men and the Goddess: Feminine Archetypes in Western Literature*. Rochester, Vt.: Park Street Press. 1990.

Bly, Robert. *Iron John: A Book About Men*. New York: Random House. 1990.

Keene, Sam. *Fire in the Belly: On Being a Man*. New York: Bantam Books. 1991.

Raines, Howell. *Fly Fishing Through the Midlife Crisis*. New York: William Morrow and Company, Inc. 1993.

Miscarriage

Allen, Marie, Ph.D., and Shelly Marks, M.S. *Miscarriage: Women Sharing from the Heart*. New York: John Wiley & Sons, Inc. 1993.

Davis, Deborah L., Ph.D. *Empty Cradle, Broken Heart: Surviving the Death of Your Baby*. Golden, Colo.: Fulcrum Publishing. 1991.

Personal Transformation

Becker, Ernest. *The Denial of Death*. New York: Macmillan Publishing Co., Inc. 1973.

Gould, Roger, M.D. *Transformations—Growth and Change in Adult Life.* New York: Simon & Schuster. 1978.

Sheehy, Gail. *Passages: Predictable Crises of Adult Life.* New York: E.P. Dutton & Co. 1974.

Viorst, Judith. *Necessary Losses: The Loves, Illusions, Dependencies and Impossible Expectations That All of Us Have to Give Up in Order to Grow.* New York: Simon & Schuster. 1986.

Relationship Issues

Beattie, Melody. *Codependent No More.* Center City, Minn.: Hazelden. 1987.

Colgrove, Melba, M.D., Harold Bloomfield, Ph.D., and Peter A. Mc-Williams. *How to Survive the Loss of a Love.* New York: Bantam. 1967.

Gray, John. *Men Are from Mars, Women Are from Venus.* New York: Harper-Collins. 1993.

Halper, Howard, Ph.D. *How to Break Your Addiction to a Person.* New York: Bantam Books. 1983.

Hendrix, Harville. *Getting the Love You Want.* New York: Random House. 1989.

Norwood, Robin. *Women Who Love Too Much.* New York: Pocket Books. 1986.

Woititz, Janet, Ed.D. *Struggle for Intimacy.* Pompano Beach, Fla.: Health Communications, Inc. 1985.

Sexual Abuse

Bass, Ellen and Laura Davis. *The Courage to Heal: A Guide for Survivors of Child Sexual Abuse.* New York: HarperCollins. 1988.

Miller, Alice. *Thou Shalt Not Be Aware: Society's Betrayal of the Child.* New York: New American Library. 1986.

Woititz, Janet, Ed.D. *Healing Your Sexual Self.* Deerfield Beach, Fla.: Health Communications, Inc. 1989.

Sexuality

Barbach, Lonnie Garfield, Ph.D. *For Yourself: The Fulfillment of Female Sexuality.* Garden City: Anchor Press. 1995.

———. *For Each Other.* New York: Bantam Doubleday. 1983.

Women's Healing

Estes, Clarissa Pinkola, Ph.D. *Women Who Run with the Wolves: Myths and Stories of the Wild Woman Archetype.* New York: Ballantine Books. 1992.

Gilligan, Carol. *In a Different Voice: Psychological Theory and Women's Development.* Cambridge, Mass.: Harvard University Press. 1982.

Koller, Alice. *An Unknown Woman.* New York: Simon & Schuster. 1982.

Leonard, Linda Schierse. *The Wounded Woman.* Athens, Ohio: Swallow Press. 1982.

Rubin, Lillian B. *Women of a Certain Age: The Midlife Search for Self.* New York: Harper & Row. 1979.

Sheehy, Gail. *Menopause: The Silent Passage.* New York: Pocket Books. 1993.

Steinem, Gloria. *Revolution from Within: A Book of Self-Esteem.* Boston: Little, Brown and Company. 1992.

Zweig, Connie, ed. *To Be a Woman: The Birth of the Conscious Feminine.* Los Angeles: Jeremy P. Tarcher, Inc. 1990.

Women's Health

The Boston Women's Health Book Collective. *The New Our Bodies, Ourselves.* New York: Simon & Schuster. 1984.

Northrup, Christiane, M.D. *Women's Bodies, Women's Wisdom: Creating Physical and Emotional Health and Healing.* New York: Bantam Books. 1994.

Appendix 3

Resources:

Organizations

Alcohol and Drug Abuse

Adult Children of Alcoholics (ACA)
P.O. Box 3216
Torrance, CA 90510
(310) 534–1815

Alateen and Al-Anon Family Groups
1600 Corporate Landing Parkway
Virginia Beach, VA 23454–5617
(800) 356–9996

Alcoholics Anonymous (AA)
P.O. Box 459
Grand Central Station
New York, NY 10163
(212) 647–1680

Women for Sobriety
P.O. Box 618
Quakertown, PA 18951
(800) 333-1606

Eating Disorders

Anorexia Nervosa and Related Eating Disorders (ANRED)
P.O. Box 5102
Eugene, OR 97405
(541) 344-1144

National Association of Anorexia Nervosa and Associated Disorders (ANAD)
1920 Thornton Lane
Riverwoods, IL 60015
(847) 831-3438

Overeaters Anonymous (OA)
World Services Office
P.O. Box 44020
Rio Rancho, NM 87174-4020
(505) 891-2664

Incest

Survivors of Incest Anonymous (SIA)
P.O. Box 21817
Baltimore, MD 21222-6817
(410) 282-3400

Victims of Incest Can Emerge Survivors in Actions (VOICES)
Voices in Action, Inc.
P.O. Box 1448309
Chicago, IL 60614
(312) 327-1500

For information on additional groups:

Organization Directory

National Mental Health Consumers
Self-Help Clearinghouse at the Mental Health Institute of
Southeast Pennsylvania
311 S. Juniper St., Suite 1000
Philadelphia, PA 19107
(800) 553-4539 Ext. 3

National Registry of Certified Group Psychotherapists
25 E. 21st Street, 6th fl.
New York, NY 10010
(212) 477-1600

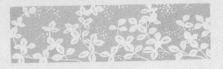

Index